DYNAMIC REALITIES
and
DIVINE LOVE HEALING

Removing Elephants from the Room

Robert G. Fritchie

World Service Institute
Knoxville, Tennessee

ISBN 978-0-9976905-1-4

Fritchie, Robert G.
Dynamic Realities and Divine Love Healing
Removing Elephants from the Room

March 2018

1. Mind and body. 2. Spirituality. 3. Spiritual Healing.
4. Self-Healing Techniques. 5. Self-Help Techniques.

Table of Contents

The Journey Map

A journey map shows the preferred route to a destination. To begin our journey, we need to define some terms.

The "*Dynamic Realities*" referred to throughout this book include amazing examples seen in our world. These are emphasized because we need to understand that REALITY is what we observe or believe exists at a point in time. A Reality can be changed and become "dynamic."

Why change an existing reality? While some people are content with their current realities, many wish and pray for improvements, perhaps to attain better food and water, improved health or greater happiness.

To *dynamically change* an existing reality may stretch our belief systems because we may not have a complete understanding about something, yet we desperately want or need to change a situation. The basic mechanism to change a reality is through the correct use of Divine Love Healing.

Unfortunately, ignored or unrecognized problems need to be resolved before we can move forward on the journey to attain a new *Dynamic Reality*. The problems may exist in various forms and at various times throughout our lives, hindering our progress. *This is the elephant in the room!*

The Cambridge Dictionary offers this simple definition of "Elephant in the Room":

"If you say there is an elephant in the room, you mean that there is an obvious problem or difficult situation that people do not want to talk about."

Dynamic Realities and Divine Love Healing

The *elephant in the room* is the *problem* preventing us from changing a static reality to a **Dynamic Reality**.

We must strive to understand how to change realities at will. This is our preferred destination in **Dynamic Realities and Divine Love Healing**.

We need to identify and begin **Removing Elephants from the Room.** In this book you will discover a journey map with which to achieve change and create your new dynamic reality.

Preface

A *Divine Love Group Healing Process* was originally taught by me in workshops. This Process consisted of a group of people sitting in a circle with the intended recipient of the healing in the center of the circle. The recipient would say a *Petition* stating what he desired to correct while the group sent the recipient Divine Love. Usually the recipient would be healed during the meeting or shortly thereafter. This successful system enabled us to obtain about 26 years of experience teaching large groups.

In 2009, we brought the *Divine Love Group Healing Process* to the Internet to teach the *Process* on webinars. Our webinars are online audio/visual presentations that enable attendees to watch and interact with me in real time. We also introduced distance healing, since our recipients and wonderful Healing Group volunteers could be located anywhere in the world. The results were the same, with recipients of Divine Love often healed during the webinar or shortly thereafter.

In 2010, as the energy of Divine Love increased in frequency throughout the universe, my life and the lives of many others were changed forever.

This book describes how our latest healing Protocols were developed and implemented. *The At Oneness Healing System Advanced Protocol* is being used today to heal drug and alcohol addiction and many other illnesses. Read, study, and share this information with your relatives and friends.

Dynamic Realities:
Overview

This book is quite different from what I have previously written. It reveals key situations that represent *elephants in the room* and describes how to correct problems before you encounter that raging herd of elephants.

In 1980 when I first investigated subtle energies most of my students thought what was being taught bordered on "magic." What they were experiencing was a Dynamic Reality that, once mastered, became a routine "non magic" healing practice.

In this book you will be exposed to many

Dynamic Realities and Divine Love Healing

"Dynamic Realities." You will learn about the true reality of spiritual healing and how we can interact with the Divine Source of all things.

Before I show you how to change your reality with Divine Love, I would like to share some information from the scientific community. Scientists have been rethinking what *reality* means. The examples shown are presented in a non-technical manner; you will quickly grasp their significance.

Learning about these scientific realities will help you understand that the concepts we are going to examine regarding Divine Love applications are REAL. What is even more important is that you will learn how to apply our energy healing principles to improve your life and health.

About Human Nature

Historically, people are reluctant to change

their beliefs. We have all heard how, centuries ago, people believed the earth to be flat and that they could fall off the edge if traveling too far. It is natural to be suspicious of anything that is new or unknown. This chapter should open your eyes to Dynamic Realities that are changing the future of mankind.

Imaginary Numbers

For hundreds of years scientists have developed complex mathematical equations to explain observed phenomena. Those equations often produced two solutions based upon what mathematicians call *real* and *imaginary* numbers. When scientists could not determine a use for *imaginary* number solutions, the solutions were frequently disregarded.

Yet, today, we find scientists using *imaginary numbers* to help explain mathematically how *free energy can be extracted from space!* This is an example of a Dynamic Reality.

Twin Particles

In Switzerland, an international team of engineers and scientists has built an apparatus called a particle accelerator to study atomic particles. A particle is placed in the accelerator and more than 9000 electromagnets develop a magnetic field that propels a single particle around a "race track" that extends for miles.

One of the original objectives was to study a single particle to see what happened as it was subjected to higher and higher voltages and magnetic fields. Although the team had developed theories about the results, they were unprepared for what actually did happen!

During one test, when the particle was slowly accelerated, all they observed was ONE particle. However, when the power to the magnetic field was increased, a SECOND twin particle appeared, and when the power was increased even further, the system overloaded, destroying millions of dollars' worth of equipment!

The physicists struggled to understand this *twin phenomenon*. Some advanced the notion of a parallel universe; others argued against the data or offered other theories; and some wanted to increase the power to the replaced equipment even further, despite the previous equipment destruction.

The experiments are ongoing; you can research the status of results for yourself. As the experiments in twin particles continue, it is likely that new uses will be found that are beyond our understanding today. This is another Dynamic Reality example.

Creating Gemstones

In the summer of 1985, I visited a secure radiation test facility in California. While I was waiting in the lobby, two large mailbags were delivered on a pushcart. When I asked what was in the bags the deliveryman showed a bag full of pecan-sized white stones from a Los Angeles jewelry company.

Later, as I passed a test lab viewing window, I watched a technician place the white stones onto a tray which was then put into what looked like a large commercial oven.

I viewed on closed circuit TV as a proprietary radiation energy was applied, causing the stones to flash a bright light, then lose their white color!

The irradiated stones had been transformed into beautiful transparent pale blue gemstones worth more than a million dollars! I was certainly surprised! This is a Dynamic Reality.

Gold From Glass

As an example of an another alternate reality, I would like to share with you an amazing discovery my dear friend, Dr. John Milewski, made years ago. John is now retired from a U.S. National Laboratory; he holds several patents.

John enjoys science and is always interested in

understanding how things work. One day at his New Mexico home, he was showing me his plant experiment to produce sunflowers more than 10 feet tall. I also noticed a huge pile of abandoned microwave ovens stacked against the wall.

John said he had always been curious about the Philosopher's Stone, an ancient method of changing naturally occurring elements into gold. I don't know where he got the idea, but he decided to bombard empty glass soda pop bottles with microwaves. When he microscopically examined the resulting mass, he discovered that the normal elements in the molten glass went through a transformation. He observed microscopic particles of gold where previously none had existed!

Although John moved on to other projects, the person who had taken over the project was threatened if he did not stop trying to make a commercial production system.

To my knowledge, the project was abandoned when the element conversion to gold apparently alarmed an unidentified industry. The opportunity to further apply this *Dynamic Reality* to other materials will be lost unless further application research is initiated.

We can say with conviction that Dr. Milewski proved that when elements are correctly stimulated, they can be changed!

This is another Dynamic Reality that I wanted you to know about.

Liquid Crystal Transformations Using Human Thought

Dr. Marcel Vogel had a patent on liquid crystals. One of the fun things I observed was his making photographs for Christmas gifts. That may not seem unusual, but it was!

While using an elaborate microscope with a camera attached, he focused on a liquid crystal specimen. He would hold in his mind an image of something and it would appear in the crystalline solution. Then he would take a color photo!

That Christmas my gift was an enlarged liquid crystal photo of Casper the friendly ghost! This is another Dynamic Reality example.

Human Cell Transformations

In the 1980's, Dr. Marcel Vogel, myself, and others regularly demonstrated that diseased cells in the body could be returned to normal. This was called "crystal healing" or "spiritual healing." This is also a Dynamic Reality.

You will see much of what we discovered throughout this book. You will also be introduced to something that has taken me on a thirty-year journey to perfect. I am talking about our *At Oneness Healing System Advanced Protocol.* When people use this Divine Love healing system correctly, they can achieve tremendous improvement in the state of their health. To me this is the ultimate Dynamic Reality and I am happy to share it with you.

Divine Love

With such an abundance of information on every subject today, people can become over-whelmed trying to determine what is real and what is not real. When people have life-threatening diseases, stress and fear may block the ability to understand the *reality* of some-thing that cannot be seen, particularly a healing system based upon the spiritual, namely Divine Love.

With my technical background in chemical engineering and aerospace, it took me years to realize just how little I really knew about subtle energies. I do understand the resistance and reluctance of scientists to study and include spiritual solutions as part of our physical reality.

What appears in front of us may represent a limited belief about the Divine. Some scientific investigators deny the existence of the energy of Divine Love and instead promote a variety of scientific terms, such as "universal field" to describe the creative force of the universe. And often there is reluctance in the scientific community to explore unexplained results, a different theory, or a *Dynamic Reality*.

Many books on the market today promote each author's interpretation of Divine Love, the energy of God's love. In addition, many books in the healthcare field offer solutions to health problems. The solutions may depend upon certain foods, medications, supplements, or herbs, as well as a host of non-conventional medical solutions involving light, oxygen, or high frequency energy applications. Some of the solutions being promoted work; others do not.

Dynamic Realities and Divine Love Healing

Someone investigating a solution for an illness is faced with an abundance of information. Major questions concerning a solution need to be asked and answered:

What are the success rates?
What are the actual costs?
Who will pay for the proposed treatment solutions?

One problem is that many illnesses as yet do not have low-cost or successful, straight-forward solutions. Alzheimer's disease, heart disease and cancer currently incur high treatment costs, with often incomplete results. Also, when new medical solutions are presented, the costs can be prohibitive.

The lack of awareness regarding the dangers of prescription drug abuse has led to unnecessary fatalities across the United States and in other countries as well. Existing solutions offered for drug addiction have a high cost and take a long time to implement successfully. Most cities and counties in the United States cannot afford the solutions. And the failure rate for people being treated in rehab centers is around 70%!

For the past 30 years, I have taught the public how to utilize Divine Love to heal physical, mental, and spiritual problems. We have had outstanding successes with thousands of people. That is why I believe healing with Divine Love is a Dynamic Reality.

Summary

In this introduction I have presented the concept of *Dynamic Realities* in the hope that you are encouraged to learn more about spiritual Divine Love healing.

This book examines the application of Divine Love healing to a variety of health problems, many of which are untreatable with existing medical techniques.

Dynamic Reality:
Religion and Spirituality

Before discussing Divine Love and how it works, we need to address some of the confusion concerning religion and spirituality. Many people find themselves restricted in their thinking because they were taught in their youth to believe in a particular religion, while the concept of spirituality was seldom discussed.

Religion

There are many religions throughout the world and I am not qualified to analyze or comment upon the pros and cons of each. Most religions believe in a supreme deity, honor nature, or revere their ancestors, with the intention of aligning man with the highest ideals.

Archaeologists have discovered ancient civilizations with sophisticated building techniques that cannot be explained by today's technologists. Those civilizations were generally developed with religions integrated into daily life.

Much of history is substantiated by religious texts found in India, China, Russia, Europe and the Americas. Going back further, history exists in stone carvings, ancient symbols on cave walls, and sacred texts found in monasteries. Although most of us cannot translate these into meaningful information, there is a resurgence of interest today wherein gifted people are able to "tune in" to various sites and interpret the messages.

What emerges is a picture of religious testimonies that were the foundations for social structure. Over time these fell into disuse as various civilizations combined or declined.

As people embrace new technologies today, we see evidence that organized religion is losing its influence. Behavior seems to be more influenced by pop culture than by religious doctrine. When I've traveled internationally, churches, temples, shrines and other religious places have often been featured as tourist sites. Yet, fewer and fewer people attend services representative of organized religion today.

Many individuals function without regard for the health and well-being of their fellow man. We see this in the Middle East, some African nations, and even in so-called "civilized" nations, where power is often wielded at the expense of attaining the higher good for all. And, we seem to have less tolerance for the cultures, religions, and politics of other countries.

Societies with many social and cultural

benefits want to hold on to what they have, while those in many emerging countries want more and better benefits.

Hope is one of the basic tenets of religion. However, as governments are confronted with situations such as terrorism and illnesses for which there are no medical solutions, disillusionment results; hope for positive outcomes is lost.

Spirituality

It has long been my belief that we have reached a point in society where we are no longer prepared to solve the major social issues confronting us. I believe that we must learn to embrace spiritual solutions based upon intercession by, and guidance from, the Creator.

Although many may acknowledge the Creator as the source of spiritual intelligence, some believe the Creator to be unapproachable or to be feared. Thus, they are locked into believing that the Creator is unconcerned about their well-being.

Nonreligious people generally acknowledge that "something out there" affects the world and rightfully consider it an intelligence greater than themselves. They may favor a strictly scientific explanation rather than accept that they can readily interact with the Divine in thought, word and deed.

This can leave them with a mindset of their own creation, defining *spiritual guidance* as whatever it is that enters the mind. This is a terrible trap because what we become, and act on, is a consequence of our mindset. If a person believes he is intellectually superior to others, then that is how he behaves.

My parents had two different Christian religions, which eventually caused a deep separation in their relationship. Because they did not understand the importance of spirituality and Divine Love in their lives, they lost hope that there were religious solutions for their life problems and consequently could not work their way through difficulties.

Observing this, I rejected their belief systems for myself. I did have an ingrained belief in God, but no particular church affiliation. The groundwork had been laid for my tolerance toward the different and varied belief systems of others.

In my 20s and 30s, being preoccupied with advancing my career, I thought little about religion. I entered my 40s realizing that world conditions were "out of control," but I was not quite ready to ask for spiritual guidance.

My Introduction To Spiritual Realities

I reflected on what to do with the rest of my life since my efforts to date had enriched corporations, but left me feeling incomplete.

I was aware that true happiness is achieved not

with material wealth or reputation, but by helping others; however, I was unsure how to change my focus.

Although I had not prayed much as an adult, I finally asked God what I should do. The answer was instantaneous and it was stunning:

In front of my face a full-color hologram of the Great Pyramid appeared, rotating on its base. I heard the statement, "Study energy!" before the image vanished. Within weeks, I had made contact with Dr. Marcel Vogel; my life was about to change!

My Introduction to Spiritual Scientists

Although Dr. Marcel Vogel was a great scientist, he was also deeply religious and deeply spiritual, a combination I had never before seen. From the moment we first met, I recognized I was to receive his spiritual guidance.

Dr. Vogel gave me a reading list of ancient literature and showed me how to sense book content to quickly extract what I needed. These books were all spiritually based, guiding the reader to understand that the universe is in fact guided by spiritual forces.

His training program opened my awareness; I marveled at what I learned! When I had completed the reading list, Dr. Vogel sent me to talk with scientists, psychics, and medical doctors. All of the people that I visited were deeply spiritual and unencumbered by the conventional beliefs in their fields of expertise. I was blessed to have had the opportunity to meet and work with some of the greatest people that I have ever known.

Spiritual Telepathy and Angels

As discussed in my book, <u>Being at One with the Divine</u>, my faculties expanded during this time. One of those faculties was *telepathy*. In my case, Angels contacted me telepathically.

Dynamic Realities and Divine Love Healing

Being uncertain of their origin and recalling childhood ghost stories, I initially resisted the Angels.

However, my adult mind reasoned that Angel contact was good if what I learned could be applied to help people. The Angels helped me immensely, bridging the gaps in my understanding of subtle energies and of how the spiritual realm functions.

While Angel guidance has been invaluable, it actually took me several years to develop sufficient confidence in their motives. Having witnessed how people manipulate each other, I did not want to find myself being similarly manipulated by Angels.

The majority of individuals I have met, whether religious or not, believe in the ghosts of their ancestors or the Angels of God. Yet when I asked if they communicated with their Angels, most people were surprised; they did not realize they could! Simply ask your personal Angels to speak to you in words. For example, say aloud:

"With Divine Love, I ask my Angels to identify themselves and talk to me."

Sit quietly and listen. Carry on a conversation and you will learn more about your spirituality because Angels are there to help you.

When asked how my Angels interact with me, I explain that, although the Angels will answer questions, I needed to learn to ask questions in the correct manner to get dependable answers. *This occurs because answers from the spiritual realm are all-inclusive answers.* We need to evaluate what part of any answer really applies. Here is an example to help you understand this subtle point. If you ask your Angel:

"Do I have cancer cells in my body?"

The answer will always be YES because we all

have a wide variety of these cells that are *not active* if our bodies are in a state of energetic balance. If you asked instead :

"Do I have any cancer cells in my body that are an active disease?"

You will get a NO if you do not have active cancer, or a YES if you do have active cancer. The answer you get is the truth for your entire being. Be precise when you are asking because your body heals first from *soul,* then to *physical body* last.

Here is another example. If you asked:

"Is my symptom healed?"

The answer would usually be YES because your *spiritual component is healed immediately upon saying a Petition.* However, because your physical body may NOT yet be healed, you could be getting wrong input. When people get a YES, they may stop thinking clearly, latching onto that answer because it alleviates their initial fears and concerns. Then they may experience continued health deterioration because they stopped healing too soon, whether by medical treatment or Divine Love spiritual healing.

Therefore you should ask instead: *"Is my symptom healed in my soul, mind and physical body?"*

This gives you a YES or NO based on the *exact status* of your entire system. Pay close attention to this wording. You will see it again when we talk about the various ways to test for results.

My Emergence as a Spiritual Scientist

In college my training as a chemical engineer gave me an understanding of how to analyze and solve problems in a disciplined, non-emotional way. This was the physical side of my training.

Dynamic Realities and Divine Love Healing

The spiritual scientist component evolved over several years as I was thrust into situations that could not be resolved scientifically. The Angels were teaching me to learn by doing and making mistakes. I learned to use my spiritual faculties to ascertain the truth about a topic then proceed toward a solution. This was tough training as I did not have a basis from which to start. It was similar to throwing a child into deep water and telling the child to sink or swim!

Yet the further I went in spiritual training, the less I seemed to know for sure. I needed to learn how to use science and spirituality together to reach solutions that could be duplicated and taught to others.

My first five years of spiritual development were difficult because often when I thought I understood a solution, a set of complications would arise. This made it nearly impossible to clearly determine a course of action. I made many mistakes and learned from them. What eventually emerged was the first Divine Love Group Healing System. For many years this system was taught to large groups throughout the United States and parts of Canada.

In 2009, I began teaching on the Internet. The sessions were well attended yet major questions were asked that indicated an absence of understanding about spirituality and Divine Love. This led to the publication of a series of books in which science and spirituality were blended to improve self-healing systems using Divine Love.

Throughout those early years, we saw tremendous changes taking place as people recovered from debilitating illnesses. This of course stimulated me to delve deeper into how spiritual healing really works. Eventually I completely opened to Divine guidance from the Angels and the Creator.

I too had believed that healing was something solely on the physical plane, such as surgery, therapy, or medications. Eventually I learned that all healing works the same way. And, it is all spiritual in origin!

Once we learn to accept spiritual guidance, confusion disappears and healing is easily implemented.

A Physical Angel

One weekend while teaching a workshop in Malibu, California, I realized that some of the participants were feeling overwhelmed by the presentation.

During the lunch break, as I stood on a cliff gazing at the ocean, I heard someone walking along the trail. There was a pretty young woman wearing a long white summer dress; her hair was braided and hung down to her waist. We had never met.

She walked up to within five feet of me, raised an arm above her head and said: "You can do this, Bob." As she dropped her arm, I felt a blast of Divine Love energy surge through me from head to foot; it was unlike anything I had ever experienced.

She smiled, turned away, took a few steps and then vanished! I was grateful for this spiritual and physical experience because it enabled me to teach more clearly; the afternoon session was more meaningful to all.

In sharing this information with you, I hope to spare you the need to experience this same long spiritual development process. If I can convince you in this book that Divine Love healing is real and that there is nothing to fear, then you will be able to achieve healing for yourself and for others.

The largest deterrent to spiritual healing is fear; it prevents one from accepting obvious spiritual truths.

Dynamic Realities and Divine Love Healing

Spiritual and Physical Effects

It is important to understand how Divine Love healing really works because it behaves differently from what you may have been taught about healing and modern medicine. Historically, many people have died from illnesses because physicians lacked effective medical solutions.

Today, pharmaceutical companies introduce new medications designed to deal with specific ailments. Dedicated researchers explore alternative treatments using all-natural products, herbs and supplements. There are also treatments such as acupuncture, chiropractic, massage, and bio-energetic devices involving heat, light, sound, and frequency. While society is becoming more tolerant towards alternative approaches, a general lack of understanding and acceptance remains.

Our health is negatively impacted when we do not take proper care of ourselves and/or overdose with prescription medications. Medical solutions may later be compromised as medications become less effective. A good example of this is our overuse of antibiotics.

Reports indicate that the widespread overuse of antibiotics on animals in China has rendered those same antibiotics ineffective for treating the Chinese populace. In the United States, we are faced with a similar problem. The existing number of effective antibiotics is dwindling.

It seems that anytime we overuse or misuse discoveries such as medications, there are unintended consequences. Because bacteria mutate and adapt to their environments, it may be too late for us to correct the damage done by overuse of current antibiotics. The drugs may no longer be capable of neutralizing or killing intended bacteria.

Technology has given practitioners many new tools and each practitioner markets his own approach to wellness, convinced that his approach is best. It is not for me to decide the correct healing approach for anyone, but you should know how to test for the truth in order to make your own healthcare decisions.

When public awareness of health and other issues is raised, our questions increase, e.g., "How can we make more progress in solving clean water issues?"

This was what I asked myself when I first introduced Divine Love healing techniques to the general public. The answer is apparent:

We need to embrace our spiritual birthrights and learn how to align ourselves with the creative energy of the universe! Why? Because we learned that:

Once people are aligned properly with the Divine, healing is facilitated.

We also learned that Divine Love healing works well in conjunction with other medical procedures. For example, for someone taking chemotherapy, side-effects can be minimized or eliminated with Divine Love healing.

A person addicted to street or prescription drugs is capable of being completely healed. This healing can occur rapidly, depending upon the strength of the person's belief in the Creator and the desire and commitment to be well.

There are two parts to Divine Love healing:

When we say a Divine Love Petition aloud, there is an immediate response in the spiritual realm as our spiritual energy fields become aligned with the Divine and then healed.

In the second part, Divine Love healing progresses from one's Spirit into the subtle energy fields of one's body. This action may require just minutes or as much as several weeks to complete the healing.

Dynamic Realities and Divine Love Healing

Since we are working with a Divine Love Dynamic Reality, researchers need to understand what test results mean in the presence of Divine Love healing. If a healing is done right now and is followed up by physical laboratory tests, such as a blood panel, general improvements are usually seen. This is not the end of the test cycle, however; as a healing proceeds into the physical form, test results improve.

It takes time for the physical body to fully respond. Therefore, you need to know how much emphasis to place on incremental test results. We want to avoid the tendency to immediately respond with additional medication or procedures in an effort to improve test results. Unfortunately this often creates a conflict in hospital care. Since they are striving for a rapid reduction in symptoms, hospitals may over-medicate, which can lead to side effects.

Usually, the body will achieve stability within 10 days using Divine Love healing; whatever measurement you use at that point reveals the spiritual and physical truth. The body on its own cannot always neutralize and eliminate the side effects. In my experience, Divine Love healing will correct side effects.

It is not my intent to discredit the medical field. Medicine and Divine Love healing are not mutually exclusive. Each of us can decide whether or not to engage in Divine Love healing for ourselves. Please review the Healing Reports on the World Service Institute website at: https://www.worldserviceinstitute.org

You will discover many different illnesses have been corrected.

Dynamic Reality:
Divine Love Energy Applications

This chapter includes real-life spiritual applications of Divine Love. The solutions were spiritual; they could not be attained by physical means.

The Fukushima Incident

In 2011 the nuclear facility at Fukushima was destroyed by the combination of a major earthquake and a 15-meter tsunami which disabled the power supply and cooling of three reactors, causing a nuclear accident.

After the earthquake, the three operating reactors shutdown automatically, but the tsunami disabled the emergency generators needed to operate the reactor cooling pumps. This led to the meltdown of the three reactors, releasing significant amounts of radiation into the air, ground and ocean waters.

The lethal radiation from the facility was measured and reported as being sufficient to kill first responders. The resulting lethal radioactive gases reached the atmosphere and carried across farmlands, creating higher than normal levels of radioactivity in spinach and milk at farms.

In addition, more than 80 percent of the radioactivity from the damaged reactors ended up in the Pacific Ocean, where it would be extremely harmful to marine life and other animals.

Shortly after the accident, 551 volunteers joined me in a webinar to implement a worldwide Divine Love Petition. The Petition was designed to protect the people of Japan and all living things from radiation damage. News-casters were confounded because no deaths from radiation exposure were being reported. Other groups may also have performed a similar service for humanity and contributed to helping the Japanese people.

What happened was miraculous to some and a mystery to others. Although experts claimed that the nuclear industry "best practices" prevented the anticipated high death rate, few people believe that.

As of October 2017, the international World Nuclear Association reported that there have been no deaths or cases of radiation sickness from the nuclear accident.

The At Oneness Healing System

Between 2010 and 2016, I developed and tested a comprehensive Divine Love spiritual healing approach called the *At Oneness Healing System*, as described in my book <u>Divine Love</u>

<u>Self Healing.</u> Using only two Petitions, this system works well for most people to accomplish whatever is needed to correct a symptom. The development of the *At Oneness Healing System* is discussed later in this book.

My intention upon introducing this *System* was to be able to train people in about 90 minutes how to use the *At Oneness Healing System* effectively. Although results have been great, those living or working in hostile or negative environments were observed to have problems staying continuously connected to Divine Love.

Divine Love exists as an unseen energy in both the spiritual and physical realms. This is a Dynamic Reality.

Divine Love exists everywhere in a neutral state. When one uses internal Spirit and a Petition, Divine Love activates, comes out of the neutral state, and begins to correct the symptom specified. However, when a person is upset or struggling to function in an environment of negativity, he disconnects from Divine Love, and healing stops.

It became evident that we needed to modify the *At Oneness Healing System* to keep people continuously connected to Divine Love and to help eliminate other limitations to healing.

The expanded program is called the *At Oneness Healing System Advanced Protocol.* The *Advanced Protocol* contains additional Petitions and techniques to keep people continuously connected to the source energy of Divine Love. This produces much faster results and enables people anywhere to use our *Advanced Protocol* with minimal instruction.

Both self-healing systems required slow, methodical testing with volunteers before either system was made available to the public. Once testing was completed, we were ready to apply the systems to conditions that lacked conventional medical solutions.

Divine Love Addiction Healing Program

Starting in 1985, I worked with individuals in California who sought help to break their heroin addictions. Word of their successes spread and I was soon helping more people in the entertainment industry. To my knowledge, all of these people have remained "clean."

Today, drug addiction statistics are widely reported, in part because of the alarming increase in overdose deaths. Parents of dead children still agonize over how they had been unaware of any destructive behavior until too late. However, governments lack funding, programs, and personnel to effectively cope with the drug problem. This represents an enormous elephant in the room!

In April 2017, I initiated a spiritual research program for drug and alcohol abuse using the *Advanced Protocol.* What was astounding was that participants who believed in the Creator had rapid success. Those who did not believe in a Creator showed no improvement.

People with successful results fell into two groups:

Group 1 people accepted the reality of the Creator and the *Advanced Protocol* and were able to chemically detox without pain medications; heal any brain or system damage; and release underlying causes of their addictions within a week. Some individuals were able to break their addictions and experience recovery in three days or less.

For Group 2 people, unsure of what they believed about the Creator or the *Advanced Protocol*, results took longer, generally 7 to 10 days.

Note: These results were achieved without any physical contact with the participants.

Dynamic Reality:
Structuring Fluids

In the late 1970's, the consulting engineering company I worked with was hired to correct contaminated water discharged from a major steel plant in Ohio. There were no local laboratories capable of doing the sophisticated testing we needed, so I set up a laboratory and hired local scientists to run the lab. For six months we used sophisticated water testing equipment to determine precisely what was in the water so we could design a solution.

We delivered a highly successful technical solution resulting in a state-of-the-art waste water treatment facility. This experience gave me a solid background in advanced water chemistry that helped me better understand structured water technology a few years later.

In 1980, as part of my early subtle energy training, Dr. Marcel Vogel showed me how to "structure and program" water using intention. It was as simple as holding a thought to affect the water, then pulsing that thought with breath and Divine Love into the water.

Marcel clearly showed that water can store information and human thought. Today structured water is being studied by industry and private institutions for new medical applications and for use as an information storage device.

My first recollection of applying structured water to a larger body of water involved a neighborhood pond where ducks had been dying. I concentrated on sending Divine Love into the pond water with the intention of protecting the ducks, then pulsed my breath. A few days later it was reported that the ducks were well; the problem had mysteriously resolved!

Dr. Vogel invited me to attend a lecture where he revealed a major finding that is still being studied by medical researchers.

A split-screen projector compared a slide containing a blood sample with cancer cells to a slide containing a liquid crystal. I explained the event in a previous book, but because of its importance, it is repeated here.

The blood sample shown on the left side of the screen was a dark blob with rough edges and multicolored streamers of matter. The right half of the screen showed a gray-colored formless liquid crystal.

Amazingly, when Dr. Vogel pulsed love to the blood slide, the edges of the blood drop were reformed into a smooth circular shape as if drawn by a wide black felt tip marker. Simultaneously, on the right side of the screen the electrically energized liquid crystal displayed a similar black outline, but in this case it was the outline of a block numeral.

As we continued watching, light flashed from both the blood sample and the liquid crystal The multicolored streamers in the blood sample transformed into a single bright red disk and the liquid crystal displayed a solid black block numeral. We learned blood behaves as a liquid crystal (which in fact it is), and that blood can be altered by thought.

I was intrigued by this presentation, but not sure how to apply it until my Angels put me in touch with people who had advanced medical problems. I was able to do healing work with people with cancer, with lupus, and with various infections.

In each case, follow-up laboratory tests proved that these people had recovered completely. Their bodies responded, whether we called it "healing" or an "adjustment to the structured fluid" in the body. This was confirmation that the healing techniques that Marcel and I were using would produce the same healing results regardless of the symptoms.

Years later several friends told me about their pets having inoperable cancers. Up to this point, I had done considerable animal healing, but had not used structured water to help animals.

I structured and programmed several bottles of mineral water without stirring the water in any way. The program was simply, *"Send Divine Love into the water to help the animal."* I gave out several quarts of the structured water and asked each animal owner to add several tablespoons of the structured water whenever they filled their pet's drinking water bowl. I did not explain anything else about the water.

Within 10 days, they all reported improvements in their pet's health. When they took their pets to their veterinarians, there was no evidence of cancer! This experiment opens a new vista of applications.

Structured water can also be used to help people alleviate pain from injury and disease. Since we had always used Divine Love Petitions to release pain and its underlying causes, I had not previously taught the use of structured water in this application. To perform your own structured water experiment to release pain:

Pour a glass of tap water and set it on a table or counter top. Step away from the glass about 5 feet. While looking at the water, say aloud, *"With my spirit I send Divine Love into the water to neutralize pain."* Drink the water then record your results.

Marcel and I demonstrated water structuring in our workshops so people could duplicate what we taught. Demonstrations included improving the smell or taste of a liquid or fruit.

We also liked to demonstrate the effect of a negative thought in water. To do this experiment:

Place a glass of ordinary tap water on a table. Again, step back from the glass about 5 feet and look at the water. Hold in your mind a negative thought, something that really bothers you. Draw in a breath and with your intention, pulse your breath, sending that negative thought into the water. When you taste the water, it usually tastes horrible.

Next, step away from the glass about 5 feet, then pulse Divine Love into the water with the intention of healing the water; taste the water again. You should detect a significant improvement in flavor.

Structured Water and Wine Experiments

After his retirement from IBM, we began structured water testing in Dr. Vogel's private laboratory. We realized that fluids could be easily structured and programmed for many applications.

Dr. Vogel had an ambitious program, experimenting with both water and wine structuring. He built a device that circulated water through a seven-turn coil, with a proprietary Healing Crystal mounted in the center of the coil.

If we programmed the Crystal with a desired thought in the presence of Divine Love, and then circulated wine through the coil, we could physically change some of the physical properties of the wine.

We used many gallons of poor-tasting wine in these experiments and some days needed to air out the lab because the fumes were so strong! In the early work, our only test measurement was taste; the structured wine either tasted good or it did not. Eventually, Marcel discovered the operational conditions that enabled him to consistently make better-tasting wine.

A winery in Northern California had produced several years of inferior wine. The samples the owner brought to the lab tasted worse than the poor-tasting wine that we had been using in our experiments!

Marcel ran the wine through his structuring device and produced a remarkable taste improvement. He loaned the winery owner a structuring device with which to treat the winery inventory. Later that year, that structured wine won top prize in a California wine competition!

Marcel loaned a second structuring device to a major wine-making company and instructed their head winemaker how to use it. However, because the winemaker had several health problems, his body took in all the Divine Love energy, discharging the device; no energy was left in the crystal to structure the wine. Twice I recharged the device, but he was still unable to use the equipment, so the venture was canceled.

Dynamic Realities and Divine Love Healing

In Dr. Vogel's private laboratory, other structuring experiments were done concerning plant growth. Both seeds and plants were treated with Divine Love structured water, sometimes using structuring devices and sometimes strictly by intent as explained earlier. Significant improvements in growth rates were observed. You can easily duplicate these experiments with the knowledge from this chapter.

Structuring is not limited to fluids. If you use Divine Love correctly, you should be able to ensure that foods are also safe to eat, however they are produced. This is true for proteins and vegetables, any food you want to consume, including beverages.

I always use a simple Petition such as this, followed by a pulsed breath:

"With my Spirit, I send Divine Love into this food to make it harmless and nutritious for me to eat."

This Petition is a mechanism that can be used to make sure you do not accidentally ingest something harmful; it does not relieve you of your responsibility to eat nutritious foods.

Water Treatment Plant Experiments

After I had relocated to San Jose California, I learned that some of the water plants in the area were closed. The water table between San Francisco and the southern part of San Jose had been contaminated for years due to careless industrial chemical disposal.

I received permission to conduct a water improvement research project at one of the closed plants. Then I built a commercial-sized apparatus similar in design to the wine structuring device and used it to treat the contaminated water.

My water plant test project used a proprietary technique I developed to lock the charge into my structuring device; I was not using a Vogel healing crystal. I was able to attain a 5% improvement in the water based upon a single pass through the equipment.

I relocated to the Los Angeles area before my San Jose structured water plant experiment could be thoroughly evaluated. I leave it to others to explore how best to use structured water to correct contaminated water. Structured water behaves differently than conventionally treated water.

The energy in a pailful of structured water, when added to a body of water such as a pond, lake, or river, transfers its program throughout that larger body of water. Obviously, the point source of contamination, whether from chemicals, human waste, or agricultural runoff, must be stopped. Then the water can be made safe.

Do you need special structuring devices to correct large bodies of water? It depends upon how and what you are trying to structure.

During a healing workshop on the East Coast, participants asked what could be done to correct an oil spill that had coated wildlife and a Rhode Island beach with sludge oil. Our group of 50 people used a Petition to directly structure the seawater. The oil dissolved in ONE day!

Unless you are a healthy person, your structuring efforts may need to be amplified to produce the desired effect. Accomplish this by using a large group or use a properly sized structuring device.

When attempting to purify contaminated water with a crystal device, always use Divine Love and make sure that the device cannot be discharged or you will fail. Those using Dr. Vogel's structuring device in the lab always operated with Divine Love, thus preventing accidental discharge.

Ongoing Research

Some people believe that structured fluid research is not supported by good science. However, all of the work Marcel and I did was carefully planned and applied using valid scientific principles. Everyone reading this chapter needs to understand that structured experiments need to be predicated on a spiritual and scientific basis.

Structured fluids have many applications; we have just scratched the surface of its potential. Fortunately, many others are doing research projects on structured fluids with good results! For example, we need to apply this technology to damaged worldwide water supplies.

Once you have read the chapters on Medications and Treatments and the *At Oneness Healing System Advanced Protocol,* you will understand the relevance of structured fluids to healing.

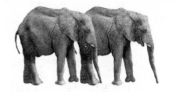 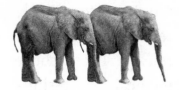

Dynamic Reality:
Medications and Treatments

Elephants in the Room

The public is generally not aware of the expense and years of research and testing required to develop new medications. For example, in a Costa Rican rain forest, pharmaceutical companies gather plant samples based upon plant healing properties revealed by local shamans. This is a commendable research effort because of the communication between shaman medicine men and scientific investigators. This type of cooperative research helps reduce product development time.

Although medical discoveries are meant to improve the health of mankind, many people are concerned with the amount and type of testing conducted on new medications before release. Those concerns are best addressed by medical professionals. Our focus is a bit different.

I have noticed some major shortcomings in the use of existing medications; these need to be addressed to avoid harmful reactions. Following are three problems that our Divine Love healing approach can help resolve.

Problem One

Those in the medical profession do not always concentrate on identifying and treating the underlying *causes* of symptoms; most treat only the *effects* of symptoms.

Medical schools do a fantastic job teaching how to apply medications and how to use lab tests to evaluate conditions in a patient's body. A patient interview and lab test results help a physician make a diagnosis and prescribe a treatment plan utilizing medications that have been shown to be historically effective.

Since most doctors do not address the underlying causes of symptoms, those underlying causes are free to manifest again when there is a recurrence of illness. *This is an elephant in the room!*

My associates and I have concentrated on the development of spiritual healing techniques that correct BOTH symptoms AND underlying causes to complement physician-prescribed treatments. No conflicts are introduced from our spiritual healing methods to compromise conventional medical practice.

Our World Service Institute website includes Healing Reports from people who have successfully implemented our healing processes on their own, without our direct involvement. Their experiences and mine have led me to conclude that:

Divine Love healing provides exactly what is necessary to correct stated symptoms by addressing BOTH symptoms and underlying causes!

Problem Two

Newly prescribed medications may react negatively with residual chemicals left in the body from earlier medications or environmental toxins. That chemical reaction can create *unidentified compounds* that remain in the body and cause side effects.

Accumulated Chemical Toxins

Pharmaceutical companies run clinical studies on proposed new medications to ensure that the new drugs do not chemically react with certain classes of other medications. Yet, it is impossible for them to guarantee that their new medicine will not react with residual chemicals stored in a patient's body. *This is an elephant in the room!*

No one company can guarantee that all medications or chemical compounds that can adversely affect us have even been identified and tested! This leads us to the obvious conclusion that some chemical reactions can produce unexpected harmful side effects. This problem also accounts for the extensive disclaimers and warnings in prescription information sheets and in advertisements. Many of those warnings have been derived from patient reports after a medicine has been released to the public.

It is reasonable for companies to reduce their liability and protect the public, but the *elephant* is still there because predicting the likelihood of all harmful side effects is nearly impossible.

Potential side effects cannot be identified until the medicine has been applied to a wide cross section of the population over time. Drug side effects may be complicated by other factors:

People with multiple illnesses may require a broad assortment of medications, some of which may interact.

Patients may not divulge all their symptoms and medications to their physicians.

There may be incomplete records when patients have received treatment from multiple medical providers.

Older persons may be more apt to have chemical remnants of old medications in their bodies.

These four *elephant in the room* conditions exacerbate the ability of even the most competent physician to get to the source of a patient's problem. For example, a physician might even prescribe a medication he would not have prescribed if he had a more accurate medical history for his patient.

If you have not fully revealed all your

symptoms, medications, and treatments to your physician, you may have added another elephant in your room and introduced more potential side effects.

I have seen many individuals with unexplained chronic pain. Often a prescribed medicine interacted with an old chemical compound already present, thus producing a new compound that resulted in their pain.

My first awareness of this problem was when I was asked by a physician to help a young woman when the prescribed pain killer had not helped. The physician ran a battery of tests, but the results were all normal and did not account for the pain. The woman had given birth by Cesarean section six months earlier and had a history of several past surgeries requiring anesthesia and medications.

Using kinesiology, we determined that her problem was caused by a chemical reaction between a drug used during her delivery and an unknown compound previously stored in her tissues.

I asked the woman to focus upon her pain with Divine Love and to release the *underlying causes* AND her pain to the Creator. Immediately, the energy disturbance and the pain left her body.

Over the years, I've been able to help many people release "mysterious" pain. Most had discordant energy trapped in their systems from side effects and drug reactions. All responded to healing in the same positive way. This led me to conclude that:

Divine Love healing can correct side effects regardless of where and/or how they originate.

Problem Three

The third problem concerns *dosage* and *duration* and applies to all treatments, including prescriptions, vitamins, other supplements, and even foods. For illustration purposes we'll call whatever is being taken a "tablet."

Following is a bell-shaped curve with a "normal distribution." The left half of the ascending curve shows how the chemicals in the "tablet" are concentrated in the body over time to attain the concentration necessary to achieve and maintain a desired symptom correction. Recommended dosage rates are defined by the drug manufacturers.

The ascending vertical component of the curve is the accumulated dosage of a medicine in a patient's body and the horizontal component is the timescale.

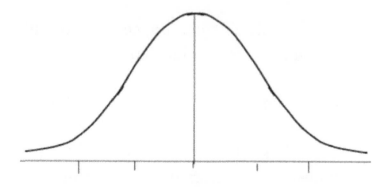

Dynamic Realities and Divine Love Healing

We would expect the peak of the curve to continue in a horizontal direction for as long as a patient continues to take the tablet at the recommended dosage. The patient would then be receiving the maximum benefit from the tablet.

However, the tablet may react with other chemical compounds already in the body, forming new undetected compounds that stimulate pain sensors. The body may also become non-responsive to the tablet, or be affected by other unknowns. Continuing to take the tablet usually produces a decline in effectiveness over time, as indicated by the descending half of the curve.

Let's apply this distribution concept to the dosage of a recommended tablet.

The instruction "Take a 5mg tablet three times a day" means that every day you would ingest a total of 15mg. Physicians follow manufacturers' guidelines to prescribe *how much* and for *how long* a tablet needs to be taken to achieve the desired effect.

At first, the graph seems easy to understand, because at the end of day 1 we would have accumulated 15mg and by the end of day 2 we would have accumulated 30mg.

However, *dosage* and *duration* of treatment are complicated by whether the active ingredients in the tablet:

Act in the body immediately, or

Are not all absorbed in the body but are instead excreted, or

Accumulate in the body until they reach the concentration needed, or

React with old accumulated chemical compounds already in the body.

Because results can vary among individuals,

multiple dosage curves may be developed and tested by researchers. For example, a drug company may recommend that a physician prescribe a minimum dose of 5mg, leaving the dosage at that level for a week or two. If the results are insufficient, the physician may then prescribe a higher dose and watch to see how the patient's body reacts.

Consider that while it is true that our tablet may be water-soluble or fat-soluble so as to readily pass through a patient's system, it is also true that the tablet may also chemically combine with unidentified chemicals already present in the patient's body, creating a side effect, *the elephant in the room*!

In our example, we would expect that once the peak of the curve is reached, the problem would be corrected by taking the tablet as prescribed. However, as this curve begins to slope downwards to the right, it can mean several things:

The accumulated concentration no longer produces the desired results, or

The tablet may be producing undesirable "side effects," or

The physician may need to increase the dosage.

All of these conditions raise interesting questions for a physician:

Is the standard graph used for manufacturers' guidelines representative of my patient, or should my patient follow a different guideline?

What is the risk versus reward? In other words, how long should a doctor observe the patient to determine whether the prescribed tablet is effective, without risking the introduction of side effects?

Are we testing to measure the effectiveness

of the prescribed tablet?

How do we know that the tablet is not interacting in the patient's body with another compound, producing a present or future side effect?

We need accurate answers to the above questions because some side effects can have serious consequences.

A physician can't always identify the *elephant in the room* because any number of compounds could introduce an unmeasurable and unidentifiable side effect. This is why a spiritual solution is needed.

Consider learning how to use a Divine Love measurement technique to answer these questions and to determine precisely what your body needs, how much it needs and for how long. Work with your physician to identify what to do for your own best health.

We will show how to test for the above problems in the chapter on Self Healing Test Techniques.

Drug Interactions

Many good websites describe what you need to know about various procedures and medications. We will examine conflicted recommendations and drug interactions for several.

The Mayo Clinic, eHealthMe, and other websites provide interesting information if you are looking for specific data. But what if neither you nor your doctors know about a potential problem?

What is the truth?

EhealthMe is a company that merges medical data from the FDA database with individual patient responses. We view the eHealthMe reports as accurate, but keep in mind that the data may not reveal all the reasons for the appearance of illnesses as study participants age.

For example, the data obviously cannot include complete medical histories from birth; dosage rates are also not taken into consideration; and we also know that illnesses may be influenced by one's age, gender, life-style, and environment.

In this section I share some reports on side effects for a number of drugs and supplements. My purpose in reporting these side effects is to help you understand how long term use of even "harmless" medications can produce unintended consequences. *This is an elephant in the room.*

Let us examine what can happen with various combinations of fish oil, metoprolol tartrate, and aspirin.

Fish oil is considered to be beneficial for the heart, helping reduce high blood pressure.

A beta blocker such as metoprolol tartrate is prescribed for heart patients to lower high blood pressure and prevent atrial fibrillation.

A small dose of aspirin is recommended for people as a blood thinner to prevent blood clots.

Anemia Concerns

I learned recently that many open heart surgery patients leave the hospital with anemia, a condition in which the blood doesn't have enough healthy red blood cells. Blood loss and other factors during surgery purportedly cause anemia.

Since heart surgery includes blood transfusions from healthy people, one wouldn't expect anemia to be an issue. If the blood didn't have anemia, then where did the anemia come from?

Metoprolol Tartrate and
Fish Oil in Combination

I queried the eHealthMe FDA database for people having anemia when taking metoprolol tartrate and fish oil in combination.

1,628 people reported side effects when taking fish oil and metoprolol tartrate. Among them, 71 people (4.36%) reported having anemia.

Of those 71, 29% were female and 71% were male. About 28% were age 50-59; more than 70% were age 60 or older. All had been on the drug/supplement for 5-10 years.

The report further stated that the top condition for nearly 41% of the 71 people was multiple myeloma, a blood cancer. Other top conditions included primary myelofibrosis (7%), pain (7%), and hypothyroidism (7%).

This strongly suggests that the body does store harmful compounds that build up over time and contribute to anemia. The storing of old medications/compounds in the body as a reason for illness is also alluded to by some cancer and Alzheimer investigators.

It is not clear from the eHealthMe report if the combination of fish oil and metoprolol tartrate produces or somehow serves as a catalyst to produce anemia and/or cancer; perhaps another drug is the *elephant in the room.*

Neither the pharmacy information sheet for metoprolol tartrate nor the fish oil websites offer any cautions about using these two in combination.

Given that Divine Love can heal both symptoms and underlying causes, are you beginning to appreciate how Divine Love healing might help you to avoid some negative drug interactions?

Aspirin Concerns

Because aspirin is a blood thinner, patients need to know from their physicians what a safe dosage is. To learn whether metoprolol tartrate and aspirin, or aspirin and fish oil produced side effects, I ordered two additional reports.

Metoprolol Tartrate and Aspirin in Combination

A report for males age 78 (+/-5) years states that the data came from FDA reports with a 48,494 person sample size. Again, specific dosage is not included.

The most common side effects with long-term use of metoprolol tartrate:

Acute Myocardial Infarction
Anemia
Bradycardia
Breathing difficulty
Chest Pain

Dizziness
Fainting
Gastrointestinal Hemorrhage
Hypotension
Pneumonia

The most common side effects with long-term aspirin use:

Acute Kidney Failure
Anemia
Fall
Gastric Ulcer
Gastrointestinal Hemorrhage
Hemoglobin Decreased
Melena
Pneumonia
Renal Failure Acute
Thrombocytopenia

This seems seems like another elephant in the room!

Aspirin and
Fish Oil in Combination

In a 40,983 sample size of males age 78 (+/-5) years, the following was reported for aspirin and fish oil:

The most common side effects experienced by people in long term use of aspirin are identical to the previous report.

The most common side effects experienced by people with long term use of fish oil were interstitial nephritis (the spaces between the kidney tubules become inflamed) and pancreatic carcinoma.

I suspect researchers may one day discover that aspirin, in the presence of certain other compounds, may act as a chemical catalyst to produce side effects.

If you wonder about the interaction of drugs and supplements that you take, you need to learn how to do self testing with Divine Love techniques.

Refer to the chapters on Self Healing Test Techniques and Test Applications to learn how to test yourself.

Solutions for Side Effects

I suggest we apply Divine Love healing to ourselves so that we do not suffer unnecessary side effects. The potential for long term illness may or may not be attributed to the interaction and retention of medications taken from childhood to present day.

Chemical Soups

Hospital patients are often given several medications in a cup to be taken at one time; this might occur several times a day. However, could mixing medications together inadvertently be harmful?

In light of what you have just learned about

drug interactions, are you comfortable with taking all of your medications and supplements together? Without self testing to know what is best, you may be introducing another *elephant into the room!*

Open Heart Surgery Problems

Open heart surgery is a complex procedure and the medical staff involved are highly competent people. During open heart surgery, the breastbone is divided in half so the surgeon can access the heart. The patient is then connected to a heart-lung machine, which completely takes over the function of the heart and lungs.

The medications given during and following surgery can produce insulin resistance, potentially resulting in diabetes. During hospitalization, a patient's blood sugar level is closely monitored; insulin is administered as needed to maintain blood sugar levels.

One would expect only compatible medications to be administered together, but this does not appear to be the case. This seems to be another *elephant in the room.*

While current medical treatment protocols may meet short-term medical objectives, is it possible that researchers need to re-evaluate these protocols to avoid long-term side effects?

Hospital Procedures

Anesthesia hampers normal breathing and stifles the urge to cough. Also, after surgery, it's common for mucus to build up in the lungs. Patients recovering from open heart surgery are encouraged to cough to expel mucus; following surgery another medication is given to induce coughing. However, because of the surgery, that coughing is painful for patients.

I witnessed a case where four physicians in the same day declared a patient's lungs to be clear, and yet the cough-inducing medication was still given. The patient was forced to cough reflexively with significant pain, without raising any mucus. This raises two questions:

What produces the mucus and how can it be minimized?

Are hospital staffs sufficiently responsive to their own physician reports?

IV Protocols

After open heart surgery, it is important to keep fluids controlled to help reduce peripheral edema. Of course, more IVs need to be inserted following surgery. An interesting procedure, since without enough fluids in the body there is a natural tendency for veins to collapse. I've witnessed nurses struggle to find a good vein in which to insert an IV; in one case it took nine attempts to place the IV.

Patients have even been given unnecessary medications through IVs when nurses are just "following orders."

Post Hospital Problems

Patients may leave a hospital with side effects not present upon admission, e.g., problems associated with blood pressure, insulin resistance, anemia, IV site infections, and sinus conditions. *More elephants in the room!*

It may be impossible for physicians to fully evaluate potential interactions between *old stored compounds* in a patient's body and medications to be used during and following any surgery. We obviously need to incorporate better treatments and ways to monitor them. Side effects are generally treated with more medications, which in turn may introduce more problems.

How many elephants do you want to entertain in your room?

Alternative Solutions

Why do I discuss medications and administrative practices? It is because I know that established protocols do not allow hospital staff much flexibility because of the potential for lawsuits and the need for conformance to standards.

I have great empathy and respect for nurses. Physicians should rely more on their nursing staff for patient information and recommendations. Fortunately, there is a simple solution for all of these issues:

Divine Love healing can help provide solutions where medications cannot. Negative effects can be blocked with Divine Love Petitions, with no conflict with medical practices. This is a Dynamic Reality.

Comas and Pain Correction

Over the past 30 years I've witnessed some unusual medical events such as:

* My mother once went into a coma following hospital surgery. Fortunately, I was able to help. As the side effect was extracted with Divine Love, her body bounced on the bed and she woke.

* Because of severe joint damage, I needed knee replacement surgery. At that time, I lacked the skill to heal my knees, but I did have experience in removing pain. Doctors were amazed that I was able to go through surgery and rehabilitation with so little pain medication. This was possible because I had learned to use Divine Love Petitions to release and heal the underlying causes of pain.

Divine Love is a healing solution that should not be ignored. I believe Divine Love healing should be made an integral part of surgical teams, in hospitals, and in medical practices because Divine Love can prevent or heal side effects.

Conflicted Research Reports

Over the last several years, I have been evaluating what works and what does not work in the world of medications and supplements. With an abundance of research reports being generated, it is extremely difficult for a lay person to extract the truth.

The integrity of some researchers, doctors and their organizations has been called into question. Some have benefited financially by presenting biased reports favoring corporate products.

It would be wise for you to learn how to test *anything* that affects your health to determine the truth about products or procedures. The chapter on Self Healing Test Techniques describes how to do this.

Self Healing Test Techniques

Divine Love Testing

You need a reliable test procedure that will always yield spiritual and physical truth as your body heals. In this chapter we explain how you can do simple tests that do not require any equipment. Following is an example of why you should learn to do self-testing.

Suppose your new prescription has been filled and you are at your vacation cabin, but without transportation, a cell phone or a land-line connection. You've suddenly become ill and believe you may be experiencing a side effect from the new medication.

Dynamic Realities and Divine Love Healing

How will you know if it is safe for you to continue taking your medicine?

Although we do not normally carry around special test equipment, you do have your internal Spirit with you at all times. That Spirit is capable of providing you with precise answers for just about anything you want to know about healing.

The information from laboratory tests allows physicians to apply corrective medications, monitor results, and adjust medications as needed; however, an illness can originate in your Soul, the energy of which cannot be measured by conventional means.

Since Divine Love healing is spiritual, not a mental process, it follows that a Divine Love test technique is also spiritual, even though we may be testing the state of the soul, mind and body.

My Early Divine Love Test Training

In my book <u>Being at One with the Divine,</u> I discussed spiritual gifts, such as my ability to sense energy at any distance relative to a person, place, or thing. Once I gained proficiency in sensing, my training in Divine Love healing began. The first year was a struggle because I did not understand how subtle energies work in the body.

I was introduced to several medical doctors who had *intuition* concerning patient health. It took me several months to comprehend this concept.

Because my intuition in those days was nil, my Angels exposed me to these four truths in detail:

Spiritual Intention flows from spirit into the body to make desired healing corrections.

Your internal Spirit may override your

stated intention in order to heal something in you that is life-threatening.

Your internal Spirit controls the healing, not you.

When you ask about the status of your healing, you must state clearly what specific part of your system you want to know about: spirit, soul, mind, or body energy.

These truths were revealed through actual individual healing experiences. As my intuition increased, it became evident that the above principles and other healing information needed to be in a format that could readily be taught to the general public.

I was led by my Angels through this chapter's testing techniques to learn how to get accurate and repeatable answers to questions. Here are five things you need to know:

We are composed of intertwined subtle

energy fields. These energy fields are both magnetic and electrical and can be altered with our internal Spirit and Divine Love through an act of our intention. This is done using Petitions and our healing process.

When we work with our internal Spirit and Divine Love, together with a correctly asked question, we can measure exactly what is happening with our bodies.

We offer four self-test approaches. Use whichever Test appeals to you because they will all give exactly the same answer.

You can test yourself to determine when you are spiritually, mentally and physically healed from a symptom you are trying to correct.

You do not have to worry about side effects; spiritual Divine Love healing corrects side effects.

Dynamic Realities and Divine Love Healing

Test One - The At Oneness Testing Method

Once you learn to use our *At Oneness Healing System* or *Advanced Protocol* correctly, you will attain an energetic level in which you are at one with the Creator. This means that you can easily do healing for yourself or others and can get reliable answers to health-related questions.

Method

Clasp your palms together and say the following Petition aloud:

"With my Spirit and the Angels' help, I send Divine Love throughout my body and ask the Creator if my (name symptom) is completely healed in my soul, mind and physical body."

Draw in breath with your mouth closed; pulse your breath once through your nose, as if trying to clear your nostrils. Unclasp hands.

Sit quietly and listen for the Creator or your Angels to answer you. Trust the answer because you cannot be manipulated in any way.

The beauty of this particular test technique is that you are receiving answers directly from the Creator or the Creator's Angels. There is no opportunity for any manipulation because you are at one with the Creator, enveloped and protected by Divine Love. However, you must ask your questions carefully to ensure that the answers you receive apply to your entire being, not just to your spiritual energy.

If you are trying to evaluate someone else, it is most effective to build an energetic link to that person by sending them Divine Love with your Spirit as part of the test. This is done in the following manner:

Clasp your palms together and say the following Petition aloud:

"With my Spirit and the the Angels' help, I send Divine Love to (name of person). I ask that (name of person)'s Spirit send Divine Love throughout (name of person)'s body. I ask the Creator if (name of person)'s (name symptom) is completely healed in (name of person)'s soul, mind and physical body."

Draw in breath with your mouth closed; pulse your breath once through your nose, as if trying to clear your nostrils. Unclasp hands and be still and listen for the answer.

It's fine if you are not comfortable using the At Oneness Testing Method. Do not struggle with any technique or frustrate yourself by questioning whether it's real. It is real, but sometimes one needs time to adjust to something spiritually new.

Test Two - Spiritual Mirror Response

In our webinars we teach how to use our *Spiritual Mirror Technique* to build self-confidence and gain confidence in the Creator. This powerful technique adds credence to the quote: "The eyes are the window to the soul."

In our Divine Love work, we use our internal Spirit, rather than our internal Soul; Spirit is a direct and higher vibration connection to the Creator. Those who use our *At Oneness Healing System Advanced Protocol* use this Mirror Test to confirm their progress. They have been taught to heal one symptom at a time, but need to know when that symptom is completely healed before moving on to another symptom. Study the chapter on the *At Oneness Healing System Advanced Protocol* for more information.

Method

Clasp your palms together, look into your mirror and say the following Petition aloud:

"With my Spirit and the Angels' help, I send Divine Love throughout my body and ask the

*Creator if my (name symptom) is completely
healed in my soul, mind and physical body."*

Draw in breath with your mouth closed;
pulse your breath once through your nose, as
if trying to clear your nostrils. Unclasp
hands.

Wait for your inner Spirit to answer you with
a YES or NO. if the answer is YES, it is safe for
you to move on to a new symptom. If the
answer is NO, simply wait a few hours and test
again.

This test prevents you from changing symptoms before your first symptom has healed
sufficiently.

Test Three - Finger Dousing

Finger dousing is a technique derived from
divining rod dousing. I once taught dousing
using rods made from metal hangers; however,
learning to use the rods correctly takes time.

It is much more convenient to simply use the fingers of your own hands. This approach is accurate, but requires that your body be in balance and that you ask closed-ended questions that can be answered by YES or NO.

Body Balance Yourself First

Many things can "knock us out of energetic balance," e.g., injury, illness, or emotional overload. Sometimes you may just have a sense that something is wrong.

Your body must be energetically in balance *BEFORE* you do any test or you might get incorrect answers. Unbalanced subtle energy bodies can adversely affect physical results.

Clasp your hands together and say aloud:

"With my Spirit and the Angels' help, I send Divine Love throughout my body and ask that the Creator balance my entire system according to the Creator's will."

Draw in breath with your mouth closed; pulse your breath once through your nose, as if trying to clear your nostrils. Unclasp hands.

In addition to balancing you for an accurate self test, this seemingly simple Petition can do wonders to relax you.

We always want to know when a healing is complete. We are less interested in specific test values, or how much emphasis to place on them because we know that specific test values change as healing progresses.

Test Method

Do finger dousing as follows:

Place both feet flat on the floor.

Form a ring with the first finger and thumb of your strongest (or dominant) hand as shown in Figure 1.

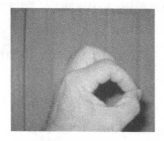 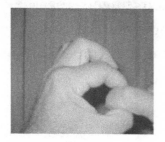

Figure 1   Figure 2

Hook the index finger of your other hand over the ring at the point where the first finger and thumb of the ring come together, as in Figure 2.

The answer you want from the dousing Petition is a simple YES or NO. If the answer is YES, then by definition it is difficult to pull the ring open with a single finger. If the answer is NO, it is easy to pull the ring open.

Calibrate Yourself for Finger Dousing

You should calibrate your finger strength before doing actual testing. This is important because stronger people tend to forcibly hold their fingers together. Ideally you will relax and hold the ring together, but not so tightly that it is impossible break the ring with your hooked finger.

To calibrate finger strength, your test answer should be an obvious YES or NO. For example, you might calibrate by saying aloud this Petition:

"With my Spirit and the Angels' help, I send Divine Love throughout my body and ask if drinking 5 shots of alcohol in 5 minutes is good for me."

Since you should know that consuming that much alcohol in such a short time is bad for you, the correct answer is NO. You can adjust the strength of your ring so that you can pull your finger through the ring by exerting firm pressure on the ring. Feel resistance without making it a strength contest; your hooked finger should pull through the ring with relative ease.

Be sure to also calibrate by selecting something that you know is good for you. In this case, you should *not* be able to pull your hooked finger through the ring because the answer is YES.

Testing

Your inner Spirit will usually answer you with a YES or NO. If the answer is YES, it is safe for you to move on to a new symptom. If the answer is NO, simply wait a few hours and test again.

This Finger Dousing Test also prevents you from changing symptoms before your first symptom has healed sufficiently.

A caution:

People using this technique frequently make wrong assumptions about the answers they receive, believing what supports their personal desires or expectations rather than the truth.

The correct way to ask a question is to include your entire being. If you are vague, the answer may apply to only part of your system and be only part of the true answer. Here is a proper format for a question:

"With my Spirit and the Angels' help, I send Divine Love throughout my body and ask the Creator if my (name symptom) is completely healed in my soul, mind and physical body."

A YES will mean that the answer applies to your *entire system.*

Test Four - Knowing

This test does not require the use of Petitions or dousing. It is a spiritual gift that comes from the Creator and is given to those who need the gift.

"Knowing" is a sacred trust that is not to be violated. If you possess this gift, you are able to look at someone and simply "know" how to help. It does not give the right to snoop into someone's private life. I only use *knowing* to help identify the source of a problem or its underlying cause.

I have met several highly spiritual medical doctors who were unaware of their gift of *knowing*. They believed their "intuition" to be a result of their experience and medical studies. In reality, their knowing came from a high spiritual source, as evidenced by their diagnostic accuracy and chosen treatments.

Correctly Wording Petitions

Again, people using these test techniques frequently make wrong assumptions about the answers they receive, believing what supports their personal desires or expectations rather than the truth.

The correct way to ask a question is to include your entire being. With a vague question, the answer may apply to only part of your system and be only part of the true answer. Here is the proper format for a question:

"With my Spirit and the Angels' help, I send Divine Love throughout my body and ask the Creator if my (name symptom) is completely healed in my soul, mind and physical body."

A YES means that the answer applies to your entire system.

If you use this *incorrect* format instead:

"With my Spirit and the Angels' help, I send Divine Love throughout my body and ask the Creator if my (name symptom) is completely healed."

You may get a YES answer, *but,* if you accept YES as your complete answer and move on to something else, you would be wrong to do so. The answer might apply only to your *soul,* or only to your *mind,* or only to your physical *body.* The wording is important!

Other Tests

What else can you test? Anything that is for the higher good and does not intrude on someone else's privacy. For example, you can test which supplements are best for you in conjunction with other medications you may be taking.

If I want to know whether taking a fish oil supplement would help my system, I would do this Petition:

"With my Spirit and the Angels' help, I send Divine Love throughout my body and ask the Creator if I should take fish oil to help my soul, mind and physical body."

If the answer is NO, it means this particular fish oil would not be helpful for some reason; more testing may be necessary.

If the answer is YES, I would then establish the *dosage* by saying:

Dynamic Realities and Divine Love Healing

"With my Spirit and the Angels' help, I send Divine Love throughout my body and ask the Creator if I should take 100mg once a day of this fish oil to help my soul, mind and physical body."

If the answer is YES, it is an incomplete answer until higher dosages have been tested.

Here is the subsequent test:

"With my Spirit and the Angels' help, I send Divine Love throughout my body and ask the Creator if I should take 100mg twice a day of fish oil to help my soul, mind and physical body."

With this progressive testing, the right dosage and frequency will eventually be identified. Periodic re-testing is recommended.

Dynamic Reality:
The At Oneness Healing System

Introduction

The content of this healing system was developed over many years from individual cases that required specially constructed Petitions to correct illnesses. *The At Oneness Healing System* enables a participant to implement a self-healing system without relying upon group support.

This healing system is based upon building a relationship between the participant and the Creator of the universe, a relationship that goes beyond conventional prayer.

Dynamic Realities and Divine Love Healing

In early 2010, we noticed that the energy of Divine Love had begun to increase. This energy increase continued until October, 2012, at which time it stabilized. We had known for many years that some individuals were capable of developing sufficient energy to function without group support. Since Divine Love energy has increased, people can learn to work independently with the Creator's Divine Love.

An interesting question was raised by a close friend: "If Divine Love does everything, why do you need to use Petitions?"

There are two reasons for my developing Petitions and healing systems. The first is that people benefit from the discipline presented in Petitions; it helps them better understand and become responsible for their own wellness. It is not sufficient to merely recite a Petition; a participant needs to understand the spiritual basis of Petitions to receive the full benefit of our healing systems.

The second reason for using Petitions is more subtle. We all experience life through a set of filters that exist based upon our belief systems and what we think is real. False beliefs and unloving behavior prevent us from attaining true Divine Love healing.

We evolve once we learn to apply Divine Love spiritual principles in ways we can relate to and believe. There are two principles upon which the *At Oneness Healing System* is based. We are given complete access to work with the Creator's Divine Love when we:

Believe in and love our Creator, and

Recognize and accept that Divine Love and Divine Love spiritual healing are real.

For example, the two healing systems that you are about to study contain Petitions. A Petition is more than a prayer. A Petition is an interactive method of communicating with the Creator. You initiate the release of a *symptom* to the Creator and ask the Creator to heal any damage caused by your symptom. When we say aloud a Petition, we acknowledge that the help being given is from a Divine source.

Components of the
At Oneness Healing System

In June, 2010, we began a 40-month spiritual research program with volunteers to test a variety of Petitions in one-on-one healing sessions. Our first objective was to develop the best method of teaching people to work independently with Divine Love. During our research, we observed that participant illnesses were becoming more complex. Our second objective was to account for and correct, where possible, anything that prevented healing.

Two of the Petitions we tested produced excellent results and they were introduced in the *At Oneness Healing System Webinar* series in November, 2013. The two Petitions were thoroughly discussed in my two books, <u>Being at One with the Divine</u> and <u>Divine Love Self Healing - The At Oneness Healing System</u>.

Following is a summary on the use of the two Petitions:

The At Oneness Petition

The *At Oneness Petition* was developed to handle a wide assortment of spiritual problems. Over time, this Petition could heal ALL root causes of energetic issues in your body. It includes a gentle release of fears, hate, forgiveness issues, false beliefs, mental blocks, subconscious issues, and negative emotional energy from others, as well as other unresolved emotional conflicts.

If it were the only Petition used, a participant could eventually recover from their illness. However, it might take longer to heal because this Petition clears multiple life-threatening problems as they occur.

Petition Format - At Oneness Petition

In the original release of this Petition, a participant would say aloud:

"With my spirit, I focus Divine Love throughout my system. I surrender my entire being to the Creator. I ask my spirit to identify every situation and every cause that separates me from the Creator and release to the Creator all of those situations and causes. I ask that the Creator heal my system according to Divine will."

Draw in breath with your mouth closed; pulse your breath once through your nose, as if trying to clear your nostrils.

The Lovingness Petition

Because most people wanted to have faster results when healing a *symptom*, we introduced the *Lovingness Petition*. The *Lovingness Petition* was designed to release and heal any *unloving* actions as well as spiritual, emotional, physical health, and life problems. The Petition uses a *symptom* to describe the problem, such as "a headache" or "loss of job."

Petition Format – Lovingness Petition

The original format was:

"I release my (name one symptom) to the Creator and ask that the condition be healed."

Draw in breath with your mouth closed; pulse your breath once through your nose, as if trying to clear your nostrils.

While this Petition works very well, there are cases where people need *both* emotional and physical healing. Emotional healing is based upon correcting unlovingness towards oneself, other people, and the Creator; this Petition was expanded to say aloud:

"With my spirit and Divine Love, I accept Divine Love throughout my entire system. I

focus on all the causes of (name one symptom) and all the causes of unlovingness towards myself, creation and the Creator and release all of the causes to the Creator and ask that the condition be healed according to Divine will."

Draw in breath with your mouth closed; pulse your breath once through your nose, as if trying to clear your nostrils.

These changes improved healing for people experiencing deep-seated emotional distress.

When a person has a single problem, this revised Lovingness Petition acts quickly. Webinar participants sometimes experienced correction of unspecified problems that resulted in removal of pain without the need to specify a symptom. This effect occurred because Divine Love heals potential life-threatening symptoms before they manifest as an illness we recognize.

As a result, some participants thought that

nothing had happened because their specified symptom might remain unchanged after several days. Eventually, their original symptom would usually heal.

This two-Petition *At Oneness Healing System* using the *At Oneness* and *Lovingness Petitions* together works extremely well for individuals living in *non-hostile* environments. Amazingly, some webinar attendees recovered from debilitating illnesses almost immediately, usually within 10 days.

Some individuals did not have good results. We discovered that they lived or worked in hostile or negative environments, with unloving thoughts, words, or deeds. Negative environments compromise healing.

Development of the
Staying Connected to Divine Love Petition

When someone is upset, feels unloved, or is unloving, that person disconnects from Divine

Love. Healing stops and the person remains in that condition until he reconnects to Divine Love. Then Divine Love healing can resume.

To keep people connected to Divine Love spiritually so that they could heal, we asked each webinar attendee to repeat our *At Oneness Petition* and the *Lovingness Petition* multiple times during the day. This was done to prevent them from disconnecting from Divine Love, because whenever a person says a Divine Love Petition, he automatically connects to Divine Love. Then healing continues based upon the objective stated in the Petition.

This summary of one participant's experience will help you understand the effects of a negative environment:

This participant contacted me because she was not getting results with the *At Oneness Healing System*. Every day she became overly stressed, even though she used her *At Oneness Healing System Petitions* before breakfast, at lunchtime, and upon arriving home.

She claimed that people in her office would badger her all day with requests for help. She would close her door at noontime and do her Petitions. Before supper, she would do her Petitions a third time.

I suspected that she was disconnecting herself from Divine Love and suggested that we talk the next day after she arrived at her office. She was connected to Divine Love at first, then, distracted by a colleague's question, she immediately disconnected from Divine Love! If she disconnected within 5 minutes of saying her Petitions, she would only have had 15 minutes of actual healing for the day!

I explained that our Healing System is a way of life that necessitates always operating in a loving way to stay connected to Divine Love, especially when working in a stressful or negative environment such as hers.

I gave her a modified Petition called *Staying Connected to Divine Love* and told her to say this Petition aloud immediately after talking with people so that she could quickly reconnect herself to Divine Love.

Disconnection from Divine Love happens when the brain and consciousness react to unloving thoughts, words and/or deeds. People are often not aware of the situation causing the disconnect.

Petition Format -
Staying Connected to Divine Love Petition

Clasp hands. Say this Petition aloud:

"With my spirit I accept Divine Love and accept my healing throughout my entire system according to the Creator's will."

Draw in breath with your mouth closed; pulse breath once through your nose, as if trying to clear your nostrils. Unclasp hands.

Because the Petition worked for most people, we immediately incorporated the *Staying Connected to Divine Love Petition* into our webinars. The importance of this Petition is obvious as it helps people stay connected to Divine Love. However, we learned that some people continued to disconnect themselves soon after connecting to Divine Love because of their negative environments.

We needed a way to keep people permanently connected. The eventual solution was to incorporate this Petition along with four other Petitions into the *At Oneness Healing System Advanced Protocol.*

Consciousness Correction

Consciousness Correction Petitions

In 1982 I studied how consciousness affects the body. It was not commonly known that one could store a mental experience energetically anywhere in the body, and have that thought adversely affect health and/or behavior later in life. Two events gave me a fundamental understanding about the role of consciousness in human health.

While having dinner in a Pittsburgh restaurant, I noticed a couple staring at me from across the room . When they later approached my table, the woman began speaking to me. I could clearly hear the words but could not easily understand because her words were all mixed up. Instead of saying something like "The quick brown fox jumped over the lazy dog," her words came out something like: "jumped fox the dog quick brown over the lazy." She felt I could help her despite the fact that we had never met. Being accustomed to Divine guidance, I was not surprised when she asked for help.

When we met the following morning, my intuition guided me to trace with my finger the outline of her body about 6 inches away from her skin's surface. Whenever my finger-tip tingled, I was able to detect phrases *locked in space* around her physical body.

I wrote down each phrase but wondered what they meant. By rearranging the phrases I was able to produce a fairly coherent story:

It seems that a month earlier the woman had been in an argument with her husband. In anger, she had rushed out of the house and driven off in her car. The car was hit by a truck at an intersection; the woman was hospitalized.

That accident had randomly imprinted her angry thoughts into her energy fields. We worked together to reconnect her consciousness and release the imprint. This was my first consciousness correction experience.

My second consciousness correction experience involved a teenage girl. Her mother asked me to help the girl, who was flunking out of junior high school. She could read, but was unable to comprehend and retain what she had read. She would begin to answer a question logically, then suddenly interrupt herself and finish with an emotional nonsensical statement.

I determined that she was oscillating between her two brain hemispheres. A healing was done for this girl to reconnect her brain hemispheres and her consciousness.

Months later the mother told me that her daughter was doing well in school and had made the honor roll. She graduated from high school with a full college scholarship, eventually earning an advanced degree.

These two experiences in healing complex emotional cases led to the development of a six-step Consciousness Correction process using *Divine Love Reconnection Petitions.* These Petitions are used to rebuild damaged neural transmitters that interact with the subtle bodies of the soul, mind and physical body.

Consciousness is a complex energy field that involves the entire body. It stores life experiences as "programs" that can trigger unexpected behavior; there may be no awareness of how or why this happens. The cause may be a spiritually untrue program in a person's belief system, or the stored program may be a long-ago event that is now in consciousness.

These stored programs in consciousness are also responsible for disconnecting people from Divine Love when their consciousness reacts to unloving thoughts. The purpose of consciousness correction is to remove the stored programs that actually block healing.

When we disconnect from Divine Love, healing stops. We may feel as if the symptom has returned, worry that we have done something wrong working with the Petitions, or believe that the Creator is punishing us. But disconnecting from Divine Love is not our fault; it can be corrected.

In my experience, many of today's diagnosed symptoms concerning behavior can be corrected once we are balanced, reconnected, and healed with our healing system. Let me show you how to begin correcting this problem.

Background on Consciousness

It is generally assumed that logical thinkers

function primarily in the left brain hemisphere and that more sensitive, artistic people function through their right brain hemisphere. The theory is that people are either left-brained or right-brained.

With sophisticated medical imaging equipment, researchers have determined that people can also be "whole brained," using both the left and right brain hemispheres equally.

After dealing with some difficult healing cases, I determined that, in addition to the two brain hemispheres, an *active consciousness* and a *subconscious* were also associated with each brain hemisphere. The *active consciousness* is an energy field that enables us to think and function on a daily basis. The *subconscious* is another energy field that stores our life events.

Stored programs influence our decision making and our responses to life situations. Sometimes those responses result in self-destructive behavior and actions that limit our healing.

Dynamic Realities and Divine Love Healing

When the left- and right-side consciousness are disconnected, multiple personalities may appear. Fortunately, conditions such as this are correctable with Divine Love healing.

In my experience, the Left Brain Hemisphere has *Active Consciousness* and *Subconscious* components. The Right Brain Hemisphere also has *Active Consciousness* and *Subconscious* components. This means that a totally balanced and functioning human being has a six-component system with which to think and store information.

Today, many people do not have fully integrated thought processes. Several participants have described the frustration of not knowing what was making them feel bad or dysfunctional. When fully integrated in consciousness, people are able to:

Recognize issues in their consciousness that adversely affect them.

Unemotionally examine all sides of an issue. They can openly express their own opinions and are open to the opinions of others.

See an improvement in decision making.

Make balanced decisions.

Before you learn how to do this, I encourage you to balance your entire body. This ensures that your subtle energy fields are able to process changes more easily.

Here is how to do a simple petition for Body Balancing:

Clasp hands together and say aloud:

"With my spirit and the Divine Love that is within me, I ask that the Creator balance my system and my chakras according to the Creator's will."

Draw in breath with your mouth closed;

pulse your breath once through your nose, as if trying to clear your nostrils. Unclasp hands.

Chakras are energy ports at various places on the body; they play an important role in processing energy.

Integrating Consciousness

Both physical and neural energy pathways connect the brain to consciousness. When a person's consciousness is properly integrated, he is able to use both sides of his physical brain and the related consciousness energy fields as needed.

Some people are unable to think or function normally because one or more of these linkages are broken or missing. The good news is that linkages can be reconnected. We do this using *Divine Love Reconnection Petitions*.

Following is a diagram showing the six-components of consciousness when looking at the back of the head. Therefore, left-sided components appear on the left; right-sided components appear on the right. The connecting lines and arrows in the diagrams that follow show how the six components connect in a mentally balanced human being.

Fully Integrated Components

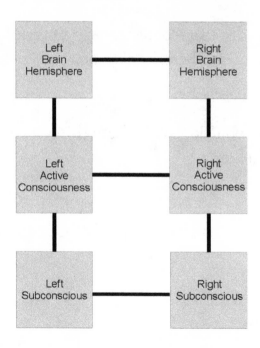

Dynamic Realities and Divine Love Healing

These six components are not fully integrated in many people, so we will begin with NO connections at all, then teach you how to build the reconnections.

As you make each of the reconnections, you may feel energy movement in your body, perhaps warmth, a tingle, or a vibration.

If you do feel something, wait until those effects subside before going on to the next step.

Even if you do not feel anything, proceed to the next step.

Go slowly and give your body time to adjust.

Step One

Connect the Left and Right Brain Hemispheres as shown by the arrows in Diagram 1.

Diagram 1

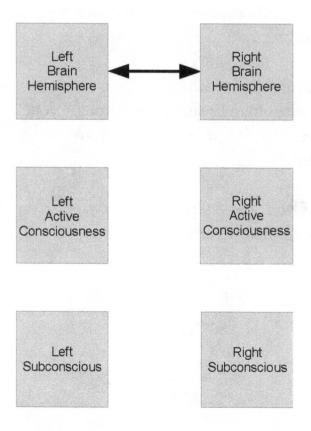

Clasp palms together and say aloud Step One of the *Divine Love Reconnection Petition*:

"With my spirit and Divine Love, I ask the Creator to connect my Left and Right Brain Hemispheres."

Draw in breath with your mouth closed; pulse your breath once through your nose, as if trying to clear your nostrils. Unclasp hands.

If you feel energy movement, wait until it stops before the next step.

Step Two

Connect the Left Active Consciousness to the Right Active Consciousness as shown in Diagram 2.

Diagram 2

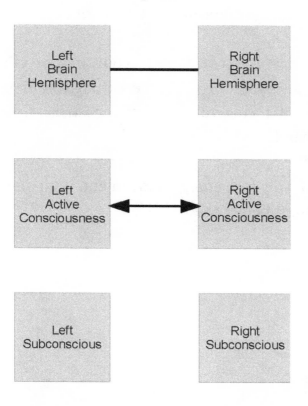

Clasp palms together and say aloud Step Two of the *Divine Love Reconnection Petition*:

"With my spirit and Divine Love, I ask the Creator to connect my Left Active Consciousness to my Right Active Consciousness."

Draw in breath with your mouth closed; pulse your breath once through your nose, as if trying to clear your nostrils. Unclasp hands.

If you feel energy movement, wait until it stops before the next step.

Step Three

Connect the Left Brain Hemisphere to the Left Active Consciousness and the Right Brain Hemisphere to the Right Active Consciousness as shown in Diagram 3.

Diagram 3

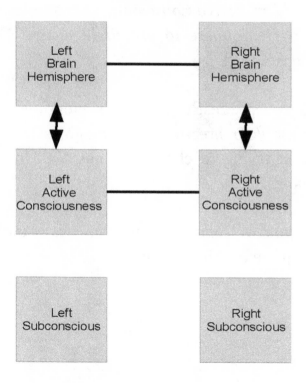

Clasp palms together and say aloud Step Three of the *Divine Love Reconnection Petition*:

"With my spirit and Divine Love, I ask the Creator to connect my Left Brain Hemisphere to my Left Active Consciousness and my Right Brain Hemisphere to my Right Active Consciousness."

Draw in breath with your mouth closed; pulse your breath once through your nose, as if trying to clear your nostrils. Unclasp hands.

If you feel energy movement, wait until it stops before the next step.

Step Four

Connect the Left Subconscious to the Right Subconscious as shown in Diagram 4.

Diagram 4

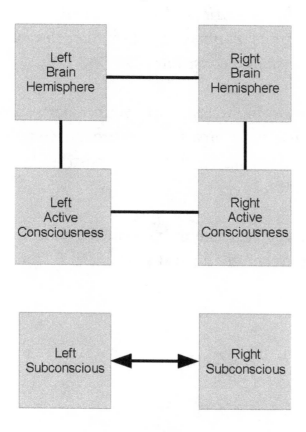

Clasp palms together and say aloud Step Four of the *Divine Love Reconnection Petition*:

"With my spirit and Divine Love, I ask the Creator to connect my Left Subconscious to my Right Subconscious."

Draw in breath with your mouth closed; pulse your breath once through your nose, as if trying to clear your nostrils. Unclasp hands.

If you feel energy movement, wait until it stops before the next step.

Step Five

Connect the Left Subconscious to the Left Active Consciousness and the Right Subconscious to the Right Active Consciousness as shown in Figure 5.

Figure 5

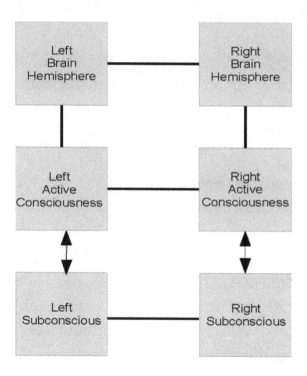

Clasp palms together and say aloud Step Five of the *Divine Love Reconnection Petition*:

"With my spirit and Divine Love, I ask the Creator to connect my Left Subconscious to my Left Active Consciousness and my Right Subconscious to my Right Active Consciousness."

Draw in breath with your mouth closed; pulse your breath once through your nose, as if trying to clear your nostrils. Unclasp hands.

If you feel energy movement, wait until it stops before the next step.

You now have a fully integrated brain and consciousness. However, we also need to integrate our spirit with our entire physical being, so that our spirit communicates with every cell in the body.

Step Six

Connect Spirit to entire physical being as in Figure 6.

Figure 6

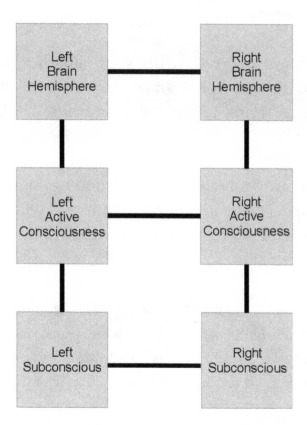

Clasp palms together and say aloud Step Six of the *Divine Love Reconnection Petition*:

"With my spirit and Divine Love, I ask the Creator to connect my spirit to my soul, my energy fields and my physical being. I accept my healing."

Draw in breath with your mouth closed; pulse your breath once through your nose, as if trying to clear your nostrils. Unclasp hands.

You are now a fully functioning spiritual being. The consciousness Petitions will run automatically to serve you for the rest of your life.

You never need to repeat this reconnection process. These consciousness Petitions are used in the *At Oneness Healing System Advanced Protocol* in the next chapter.

Dynamic Reality:
The At Oneness Healing System
Advanced Protocol

By 2016, we had accumulated significant data by applying the original *At Oneness Healing System Petitions* to difficult cases. We had also seen a sharp increase in cases of people suffering from old traumas and emotional blockages; they were prime candidates for the *Advanced Protocol.*

We wanted to expand our spiritual research programs into areas that were not currently offering solid solutions, e.g., drug addiction and Alzheimer's. We realized that these efforts would have to be accomplished with minimal instruction because many affected people do not have full control of their mental faculties.

We believed that if we incorporated the Petition experiences we had been collecting over the years into an *At Oneness Healing System Advanced Protocol*, we could help mitigate healing problems. However, the solution needed to be capable of running *automatically* with *little to no input from participants*. I felt that a three-part Protocol was needed:

Part 1 - Consciousness correction to unlock energy blockages.

Part 2 - A 5-Petition component that would support Divine Love healing under various health conditions.

Part 3 - A short Petition for an individual to communicate his needs to the Creator.

This chapter explains the development of the

At Oneness Healing System Advanced Protocol and why it is important.

Your personal *At Oneness Healing System Advanced Protocol* can be built from the information contained in this chapter.

Part 1 - Development of Consciousness Correction

Consciousness Correction from a previous chapter is Part 1 in our *At Oneness Healing System Advanced Protocol*. We have had some Consciousness Correction information for nearly 30 years, but did not release it because most participants were not sufficiently disconnected to warrant the extra instruction required.

Today, with so much chaos in the world and an increase in major drug and alcohol addictions, which disconnect people, it is time to show how to reconnect consciousness.

Dynamic Realities and Divine Love Healing

Part 1 is needed so that a person can access any area of their consciousness to release blockages to healing called *pop-ups*. We will further explain pop-ups in Part 3 of the *At Oneness Healing System Advanced Protocol*.

The physical action of integrating a person's consciousness needs to be done only once in a lifetime!

Petition Format - Consciousness Correction

Use the *Divine Love Reconnection Petitions* from the Consciousness Correction chapter to build Part 1, but only if you have not already done so as shown in an *At Oneness Healing System Advanced Protocol* Webinar/video.

Hand Placement

In this chapter you will see an unusual use of your hands when you are saying Petitions. Hand position is important when working with energy fields.

When you clasp your palms together and do a Petition, you are uniting the left and right brain hemisphere of your brain and your physical body energetically. For that reason, you are asked to:

- Clasp hands together BEFORE you start a Petition.

- Keep the hands together.

- Say your Petitions aloud, then pulse your breath.

- Unclasp your hands.

Repeat this hand clasping technique BEFORE starting your next Petition. We suggest you use hand clasping every time you do a Petition.

Part 2 - Development of the Five Petitions

By November 2016, we had completed testing five Petitions used to address most of the problems encountered during complex healings:

Resistance Petition
At Oneness Petition
Staying Connected to Divine Love Petition
Lovingness Petition
Educating Your Cells Petition

These five Petitions are Part 2 of the *At Oneness Healing System Advanced Protocol.*

Resistance Petition

We noticed that some people had difficulty releasing the events and feelings that held them back, e.g., emotional pain caused by negative experiences with families, friends, or coworkers. Spiritual misunderstandings and emotional turmoil should be released as they occur.

We had observed that holding on to old emotional wounds was a major deterrent to achieving good healing results. Therefore, we developed and tested a new Petition called the *Resistance Petition*. We determined that this Petition was useful for correcting two problems: misunderstanding our Petition content and insufficient oxygenation of cells.

Resistance Petition - Misunderstandings

Some people did not understand the meaning of some of the phrases in our Petitions. For example, the *At Oneness Petition* had the sentence, "I surrender my entire being to the Creator." The intention is for the participant to surrender *his mental effort to control the healing* by allowing the Creator to lead the healing spiritually.

Whatever the reason – fear, lack of self-worth, or religious confusion – quite a few people were reluctant to allow an unseen energy source to redirect their lives. This problem resolved when we included a clause in the Resistance Petition that says "I release to the

Creator all my resistance to healing."

Resistance Petition - Insufficient Oxygen

Even normally healthy people do not always recognize the importance of deep breathing. Some webinar participants had lung problems or were very ill and could not breathe deeply.

Deep breathing helps ensure that someone experiencing Divine Love spiritual healing is providing sufficient oxygen to their cellular structure. It has long been known that oxygen must be provided to the mitochondria for cells to live in a healthy state. Mitochondria are the components of cells that convert oxygen and nutrients into energy.

We incorporated a phrase into the *Resistance Petition* to ensure that the *spiritual essence of oxygen* was able to enter the body: *"I ask that the Creator send oxygen into my being as needed to heal my cells according to the Creator's will."*

Resistance Petition - Spiritual Essence

Our physical reality includes all we can see, hear, and touch. There is also a spiritual world that we typically do not see, but can experience as spiritual energy coming to us.

Years ago, an American Indian medicine chief taught me how this spiritual to physical transition works. I had asked how Indians were able to run for miles or hunt all day long, without drinking water. He explained that by spiritual intention, anyone is capable of bringing into their system the *spiritual essence of water.* This spiritual essence works directly on the cellular structure of the body to keep the body in balance and hydrated. I respected the chief and asked him how I could best implement this technique in my own life.

He smiled at me and said "Go try it." I decided to test this technique for myself. The following morning I ate breakfast and had one cup of coffee. With my compass and a map, I set off running and walking up and down hills near Carmel Valley, California.

Using my spiritual intention, I was able to re-hydrate my body despite the hot summer day. I sweat profusely for about four hours, then returned home feeling fine! This true story is the foundation for understanding the next paragraph.

We are able to work with our internal spirit and Divine Love to bring whatever we are lacking energetically into our systems from the spiritual realm. We can bring in not only the spiritual essence of oxygen, but also other nutrients that directly affect our cells.

This Petition is useful when people are unable to breathe deeply. Otherwise, if you are able, it is expected that you will do your own deep breathing.

Resistance Petition - Format

Clasp hands. Draw in your breath and say aloud:

"With my spirit, I send Divine Love into my entire being. I release to the Creator all my resistance to healing. I ask that the Creator send oxygen into my being as needed to heal my cells according to the Creator's will."

Draw in breath with your mouth closed; pulse your breath once through your nose, as if trying to clear your nostrils. Unclasp hands.

Development of the At Oneness and Staying Connected to Divine Love Petitions

These two Petitions are used without change from the original *At Oneness Healing System* release. Be sure to use hand clasps and the breath pulse.

Dynamic Realities and Divine Love Healing

Lovingness Petition

Several changes were made to the original Lovingness Petition to allow the Creator, rather than the participant, to specify the symptom used.

Lovingness Petition - Format

Clasp palms together and say aloud:

"With my spirit, I send Divine Love to all the causes of whatever the Creator selects for me and all the causes of related unlovingness towards myself, creation and the Creator. I release all causes to the Creator and ask that the condition be healed according to Divine will."

Draw in breath with your mouth closed; pulse your breath once through your nose, as if trying to clear your nostrils. Unclasp your hands.

Development of the Educating Your Cells Petition

I worked with several people who had become physically disadvantaged through accidents or disease and were missing signals from the brain to their extremities. In people with head/brain injuries, the swelling or physical damage could be repaired, but paralysis might remain in the extremities, or other body parts might not function properly. A Petition was developed to enable the brain to reestablish cell connections via nerves and neural pathways. Think of neural pathways as information highways between cells.

Educating Your Cells Petition - Format

Clasp palms together and say aloud:

"With my spirit, I send Divine Love throughout my system and tell all my cells that they are healed and should operate as normal cells according to the Creator's will."

Draw in breath with your mouth closed; pulse your breath once through your nose, as if trying to clear your nostrils. Unclasp your hands.

Benefit Summary for Part 1 and Part 2

Three important benefits for using the *At Oneness Healing System Advanced Protocol:*

Part 1 and Part 2, once constructed, stay in an individual's energy field for life, serving as needed.

These petitions can be set up to run automatically, without further effort on the part of the individual.

And finally, the individual remains permanently connected to Divine Love!

Part 3 - Development of the Healing Statement

We needed to make the *At Oneness Healing*

System Advanced Protocol work as an integrated healing system capable of healing specified symptoms. This was accomplished with a new Petition called the Healing Statement.

The Healing Statement is an *action* Petition in which an individual uses his spirit to release a symptom energetically to the Creator, then asks the Creator to heal the symptom at all levels of his being. This Petition also acknowledges the Creator by asking that the symptom be healed in accordance with the Creator's will because the Creator directs the healing, not the individual.

The Healing Statement - Format

Clasp palms together and say aloud:

"I release to the Creator from my entire being all my (name your symptom) and ask that the Creator heal any damage from all my (name your symptom) throughout my entire being according to the Creator's will."

Draw in breath with your mouth closed; pulse your breath once through your nose, as if trying to clear your nostrils. Unclasp your hands.

DO A HEALING STATEMENT ONLY ONCE FOR A GIVEN SYMPTOM.

Pop-ups

A person's body heals in *layers* from the outside to the inside of the body. Consider the layers of an onion. In people, the layers are the subtle energy fields, the intertwined energies of soul, mind, and body. Energetic blockages to healing can build up on these layers, with some blockages in the physical body and some in consciousness.

Once a Healing Statement is said, the body begins to heal. Healing proceeds layer by layer. If an experience or memory stored in consciousness is related to the symptoms being worked upon, healing may slow down or stop until that consciousness blockage is removed.

An example of a consciousness blockage would be someone who believes:

"I have had this illness for so many years I cannot possibly be healed."

When a phrase such as that "pops up," it prevents the body from healing; it is a blockage. Pop-ups can be memories, emotions, and images that occur to you while you are awake or while you are sleeping.

If it is important to know the specific reason for a pop-up, that information will flow to you from spirit. Or, if internal spirit does not reveal the reason for the pop-up, you may only become aware that there are consciousness issues that affect your health.

Remember that Consciousness Correction properly reunites the physical and energetic components of brain/consciousness as soon as

Part 1 runs. This gives an individual access to their consciousness so that they can release pop-ups with a Healing Statement.

Procedure for Finding Pop-ups

The fastest way to identify pop-ups is to close your eyes and take in a deep breath. This helps you concentrate. As you breathe out, go with your internal spirit and Divine Love into your entire being with the intention that your internal spirit reveal all the pop-ups that are preventing your original symptom from healing.

When you open your eyes, wait patiently and be prepared to make a written list. You may start to rapidly receive all of the requested pop-ups from your consciousness. Be sure to list the pop-ups in the order received. Each pop-up is a *symptom* that you will use in a Healing Statement.

Once you have developed a list, put the *first*

pop-up into a Healing Statement and release it. Wait a few minutes and then use the Mirror Test to be certain the first pop-up is completely cleared from your soul, mind, and body. Then proceed to put the *second* pop-up into a Healing Statement.

Here's how to do the Mirror Test:

Look into your eyes in a mirror and ask yourself:

"Is my symptom completely healed in my soul, mind and physical body?"

Listen quietly for the answer to come from within yourself. If the answer is NO, you are not healed. Do some deep breathing. Wait an hour, then test again.

If the pop-up has not cleared, wait and do some more deep breathing. Repeat the Mirror Test at one hour or longer intervals until you know for certain that the pop-up has been cleared and healed. Most pop-ups will clear within a few hours; very few take longer.

DO A HEALING STATEMENT ONLY ONCE FOR EACH POP-UP SYMPTOM.

Please use a Mirror Test to determine when the pop-up is completely released. If you do not use a Mirror Test, release and heal only ONE pop-up a day because some pop-ups may be very deeply rooted in your consciousness and/or in your physical body. Once a pop-up is removed, the body may need a few hours of rest time to recover.

An example of a deeply rooted pop-up is mental or physical abuse from childhood. Perhaps someone in conversation awakens a memory of that time you were *shamed* by a family member. Your immediate reaction is extreme anger, then frustration, as you realize that the memory of the *shaming* has triggered your anger. Put the word *shaming* into a Healing Statement and release it immediately.

Deal with pop-ups as they manifest by using a Healing Statement, then use the Mirror Test to ensure that the pop-up has cleared.

In the example of *shaming*, look at your eyes in the mirror and think about the shaming incident. Once the pop-up is totally cleared, you will be able to think about the shaming without triggering any sort of emotional response.

When you have a dream that seems meaning-less or totally unrelated to anything in your life, do not struggle to analyze the dream. If the Creator wants you to know the meaning of a dream, you will become aware of it. Because both your internal spirit and the Creator know exactly what the dream means, your only objective is to rid yourself of the pop-up. Simply use the word *image* in the Healing Statement to define the entire dream.

When you have cleared your entire pop-up list, wait a few hours, then repeat the

Procedure for Finding Pop-ups to make sure all pop-ups have been identified. This is important because sometimes when your body is healing, your internal spirit will block you from sensing additional pop-ups until the current pop-up is completely healed.

When all your symptom-related pop-ups are cleared, you will generally find your original symptom heals quickly.

If your symptom is something such as a pain or emotion, the healing will be obvious. If your original symptom can only be evaluated by other testing, then wait about 10 days to get a certified test. Most people find that their condition corrects in that time frame. If you rush to be tested before healing is complete, the test may indicate only partial healing.

The chapter on Self Healing Test Techniques describes how to test for complete healing of any symptom or pop-up.

About Describing Symptoms

We receive a lot of questions about symptoms. Here are two important considerations when deciding the best way to describe a symptom:

1. As an example: your foods seem to produce an unusual amount of intestinal gas. You might spend weeks trying to isolate the condition, eliminating foods individually or in combination, but still not obtain relief.

When confronted with a situation with many variables, it is simpler to specify a symptom that correctly describes what is happening.

In this example, if you use the symptom "intestinal gas," you would encompass all possible causes.

2. People are often prone to use a medical *diagnosis* to describe their symptoms. It is better to describe what you are *experiencing*, such as a headache, a pain in the side,

forgetfulness, or difficulty breathing, sleepless-ness hearing, or seeing. For emotional issues, use what is bothering you as the symptom, e.g., insufficient income or an unhappy relation-ship.

If you specify a symptom based on a medical diagnosis, but that diagnosis happens to be wrong, nothing happens when you use any Divine Love Petition or Advanced Protocol because you asked to correct something that you do not have!

Physical Oxygen Levels

We need to discuss physical oxygen because there has been controversy for many years over claims that increased oxygen intake will correct certain diseases. We make no claims because each case has its own requirements for healing. On our webinars we teach how to do deep breathing.

As you do deep breathing for 5 to 10 minutes, you increase the oxygen level in your blood. You can measure your oxygen uptake progress with an oximeter, an inexpensive oxygen sensing device that is placed on your index finger. It is good to maintain oxygen levels as close to 100% as possible.

Many people do not or cannot breathe deeply enough, so their oxygen levels drop. Some are averse to wearing oxygen masks or nasal cannulas.

In my experience, when the blood oxygen percentages drop to the mid 80's, a patient may exhibit confusion, fogginess, pressure in the head, inability to think, or lack coherent speech. When the oxygen level drops below 80%, people can enter into a state approaching unconsciousness. If this condition prevails, cell deterioration results. And of course if oxygen levels remain too low for too long, one can die.

Four-Cycle Breathing Technique

When using the *At Oneness Healing System Advanced Protocol,* it's important to use a deep breathing technique to fully oxygenate your cells for faster healing. Many people believe healing must follow traditional time frames but this is incorrect; we have seen many heal in just minutes! Those who heal fastest are fully oxygenated most of the time.

The *At Oneness Healing System Advanced Protocol* first produces immediate healing in the spiritual realm; that energy then moves into the physical body to correct your health.

If you do not receive sufficient oxygen, the *At Oneness Healing System Advanced Protocol* will help you through the *Resistance Petition.* However, if your spirit determines that you are physically able to do deep breathing but do not, your spirit will stop the healing process. You need to assume full responsibility for yourself and do deep breathing.

Four-Cycle Breathing - Format

Before beginning this breathing exercise, tighten your stomach muscles, pulling your belly-button in toward your spine. This compression allows more air to go directly into your lungs. Try to keep your stomach compressed in this manner throughout the breathing cycle. If you become tired, relax your stomach muscles after the 4th cycle, rest for awhile, then start again.

Cycle 1 - Breathe in deeply and slowly until your lungs are full.

Cycle 2 - Hold your breath for a slow mental count of five.

Cycle 3 - Breathe out slowly, emptying your lungs completely.

Cycle 4 - Do not breathe for a slow mental count of five.

Repeat these four cycles as often as you like.

Whenever you do a Petition, plan to spend 4 to 5 minutes doing this type of breathing. If for some reason you are uncomfortable with this technique, try slow deep breathing without holding your breath. Experiment with this to find the method that serves you best.

Symptom Healing Times

"How long will it take to heal a symptom?"

Healing time depends on several variables. For example, a 20-year-old with a headache can be expected to have a much shorter healing time than a 65-year-old with several different health problems.

Before the *At Oneness Healing System Advanced Protocol* was developed, when a symptom went away, we added three days in which you did nothing more than occasional deep breathing. If your symptom was still gone at the end of the 72 hours, it was safe for you to proceed with a new symptom.

This practice is no longer necessary; with the *At Oneness Healing System Advanced Protocol* we use a Mirror Test to validate complete healing.

When you do a Mirror Test, you are conducting the most exacting test possible. I have learned to depend on this test. If you are not yet comfortable with the Mirror Test, you may use one of the other measurement systems identified in the chapter on Self Healing Test Techniques.

Pop-up Healing Times

People are often confused by healing times when dealing with pop-ups. Here is an example to help you better understand timing and the use of a Healing Statement:

Joe has a *headache* and a *sore wrist*. To further complicate the problem, let's assume that Joe has TWO pop-ups associated with the headache and ONE pop-up associated with the sore wrist.

Here is how Joe should proceed with his self healing:

Joe says aloud a Healing Statement using "headache" as his first *original* symptom.

After a few minutes, when Joe's head stops hurting, he does a Mirror Test and learns that his symptom is not yet fully healed.

Joe does several 10-minute sessions of deep breathing several times during the afternoon.

Joe does another Mirror Test and learns that the symptom is still NOT completely healed. He then uses the *Procedure for Finding Pop-ups* and lists them. His list reveals that his headache is related to: *anger toward his girlfriend* and *frustration.*

Joe does a Healing Statement using *anger*

toward his girlfriend as the symptom and waits 5 minutes.

Joe does a Mirror Test and learns that the pop-up is completely healed.

Joe does a Healing Statement using f*rustration* as the symptom.

Joe does a Mirror Test and learns that the *frustration* pop-up is completely healed.

Joe does a Mirror Test to see if his *headache* symptom is completely healed and learns that it is fully healed.

Now Joe feels pretty confident, so he does a Healing Statement using *sore wrist* as his *second original* symptom.

After 10 minutes of deep breathing, Joe does a Mirror Test and learns that the *sore wrist* is not completely healed, so Joe decides to go immediately to the *Procedure for Finding*

Pop-ups and learns that he has a pop-up about his *low income.*

Joe does a Healing Statement using *low income* as a symptom. Then Joe does 10 minutes of deep breathing several times over the next day.

Joe does a Mirror Test to see if the *low income* pop up is completely healed. Joe learns that it is fully healed.

Joe does a Mirror Test for complete healing of his second original symptom, the *sore wrist.* He learns that it is completely healed.

From the above example, you now know how to proceed with Healing Statements, *original* symptoms and *pop-up* symptoms. It may be necessary for you to do deep breathing over many days to help your cells heal.

A more complicated situation develops if, during the healing described above, Joe suddenly experiences a NEW pain, say in his elbow. He should IMMEDIATELY do a Healing Statement using elbow pain as the symptom, do some deep breathing, and use the Mirror Test. After the test confirms that the elbow pain is completely healed, Joe should do a Mirror Test on whatever pop-up he was clearing when the elbow pain started.

How We Get Sick

In our webinars, we discuss the many ways people can become ill. Many people store negative emotions; those stored emotions are energy programs that become locked into their systems. When enough of these programs collect in the body, they are capable of blocking neural pathways and the energy of soul, mind and physical body. This causes the body to go out of balance energetically, then cells become blocked, unable to function properly.

Another way people become ill is through

physical injury from accidents; cosmic or nuclear radiation damage; and chemical damage from contaminated air, foods and liquids. Long-term toxicity from what is put on our skin can also cause the body to go out of balance and again block cells.

The *At Oneness Healing System Advanced Protocol* deals effectively with all of these conditions.

About Healing Recovery

Please do not underestimate the importance of the recovery process. Some people push themselves beyond reasonable limits even when recovering from debilitating illnesses. They want to immediately celebrate their wellness, but tend to be overactive.

What they NEED is to rest, helping the body become healthy by toning down activity levels while maintaining high oxygen levels. The Four-Cycle Breathing Technique is a proven way to raise the oxygen level of the body; it is VERY important for your well-being.

Benefits of the Advanced Protocol:

- Part 1 and Part 2 are each said only ONCE in your lifetime. Then Part 1 and Part 2 continue to serve you automatically throughout your life.

- Part 3, your Healing Statement, is the only Petition you need to use going forward, together with deep breathing.

- All *At Oneness Healing System Advanced Protocol* Petitions are directed by an individual's internal spirit and the Creator.

- Manipulation and misuse are impossible.

- If your spirit perceives that you are trying to do too many things by changing symptoms before the original symptom is healed, your spirit stops processing the Petitions so the body can recover. Then your spirit restarts the Petitions.

- The Petitions switch on and off as needed to accomplish healing.

- The individual is connected to Divine Love continuously; hostile environments are no longer a healing issue. This is because the *At Oneness Healing System Advanced Protocol* activates within you automatically.

- Once an *At Oneness Healing System Advanced Protocol* is in place, you use only a single Healing Statement said only once for each symptom.

- If any other symptoms "pop-up," you use that new pop-up as a symptom in a Healing Statement, which allows the pop-up to release and heal.

- The "Oneness" state facilitates healing.

- An *At Oneness Healing System Advanced Protocol* surrounds the individual as if he were in a bubble, acting to heal whatever single symptom is described in a Healing Statement, unless the Creator chooses to heal something more important in the body.

- When the *At Oneness Healing System Advanced Protocol* is correctly modified, it can be transmitted to the mass consciousness, where it becomes available to whoever needs it to resolve problems. This was done with our free spiritual research Divine Love Addiction Healing Program and free Alzheimer's Divine Love Healing Program.

- Deep breathing facilitates faster healing.

Teaching Aids

Webinars are an excellent way to learn all about our *At Oneness Healing System Advanced Protocol*, but the principles may be difficult to grasp and retain in a single 90-minute webinar. To relieve this problem, we offer a streaming video that can be played anytime to study or review details.

This ensures that the *Advanced Protocol* is taught correctly with the intended content, maintaining the quality level. People report that they learn something new each time they watch a video of the *At Oneness Healing System Advanced Protocol*.

Future of the At Oneness Healing System Advanced Protocol

I believe our healing system can be a great benefit to humanity, particularly when used in conjunction with conventional medicine and medical techniques. The *At Oneness Healing*

System Advanced Protocol is meant to improve the health recovery experience.

Once a participant has built an *At Oneness Healing System Advanced Protocol* or it is provided through the mass consciousness, he only needs to use a simple Healing Statement that identifies the current symptom being worked upon.

The *At Oneness Healing System Advanced Protocol* is not in conflict with conventional medicine or other proven health practices. Hundreds of people have recovered from illnesses and debilitating diseases when medical and/or pharmaceutical solutions were not available, or had not yet been discovered. However, Divine Love was able to heal.

Many individuals do not divulge their Divine Love healing experiences to their physicians. Over time, we expect that everyone will recognize the spiritual truth of this *At Oneness Healing System Advanced Protocol*, and it will be more widely shared. People will look upon Divine Love as a primary source for effective dynamic healing without side effects.

In rural areas and in underdeveloped nations, where conventional medical care is often lacking, this *Advanced Protocol* may be the only method available for healing.

The *At Oneness Healing System Advanced Protocol* provides a new Dynamic Reality to the medical community. Rather than debate treatment options, we can work together to achieve the best possible outcomes for patients, without introducing elephants into the room.

Dynamic Reality:
Test Applications

This chapter is intended to help you develop the discipline needed to learn spiritual AND physical truths.

You have learned that our work with Petitions is spiritual rather than mental. What we have not discussed is a comprehensive test for both spiritual and physical effects. The ability to do this confidently is an *alternate reality* because science has been limited to developing analytical tools.

We see reports on variables such as blood pressure, pulse rate, blood oxygenation, and measurements of some industrial and absorbed chemicals. Blood and tissue samples are used to evaluate conditions in the body. Amazing work is also being done by research chemists who formulate new microbiological and bio-chemical treatments.

But how do you measure the effect of some-thing in your system if you do not have access to a laboratory or sophisticated equipment?

In the 1980s, one of IBM's most prominent researchers, Dr. Marcel Vogel, had access to the latest in instrumentation and microscopy. His patents include the original magnetic coatings from which disk storage devices are made. Marcel was also an expert in crystallog-raphy, the study of crystal formations. He took his science background to a new level when he began exploring the spiritual energy of Divine Love.

Our friendship developed because we were both searching for ways to help people without competing with either the medical profession or the pharmaceutical industry.

Eliminating Fear of the Unknown

Because Marcel was concerned that young children were not developing their own faculties, he began a children's training course. He showed the children how to visualize and use spiritual energy to "see" distant scenes, such as what was on a faraway mountaintop.

As the children developed their skills, in their "mind's eye" they were even able to see what was happening on other planets. This included descriptions of terrain, structures, and occupants. To Marcel's dismay, when the children told their parents of their experiences, the parents did not approve and the school asked him to discontinue his course.

The great lesson from this: Doing or teaching something out of the ordinary will be met with resistance until we've eliminated fear of the unknown. People must be shown the benefits of change to accept and appreciate new information.

Development of Healing Devices

After one of Marcel's lectures, an American Indian woman asked why he had not studied crystals relative to healing. She did not elaborate, but her question resonated with Marcel. A few days later he dreamed about the physical form of the Kabbalah, and was shown in the dream that a similar physical form cut from quartz could transmit energy.

Marcel acquired some pure quartz crystals, then hand cut several into the shape shown in his dream. He gave me the fourth one to evaluate.

We learned that we could extract from an individual's bio-energy fields the energetic patterns or programs that were making him unwell. When this was done with Divine Love intention, the body would shake as it released energetically whatever caused the illness. Then we would ask the individual to do deep breathing and take in love to complete the healing.

Over time our techniques were perfected and the devices became known as Vogel Healing Crystals.

In the meantime, I had continued developing my internal measurement skills, which I consider spiritual gifts. I believe these were given to help me determine what makes people unwell. I also needed to understand the effects on the body when "bad" energy is released. This led me to an awareness of *body energy charging* and *body balancing.*

Importance of Body Balancing

I suggested in a previous chapter that you use the Body Balancing Petition to balance your body energetically before attempting a self-testing measurement. This avoids incorrect answers and ensures that your body is fully charged energetically.

Note: People with chronic fatigue are not fully charged energetically.

The human body behaves much like a battery. When fully charged, your system can perform correctly, but if depleted of energy, severe fatigue results. Once I learned how people could use a Body Balancing Petition to charge and balance the body, that knowledge became a standard teaching in my workshops.

I once demonstrated the importance of body balancing to a group of physicians. Two members of the group volunteered to have their bodies individually wrapped around in plastic drop cloths, such as those used by house painters.

Soon, as they stood in front of the group, both volunteers began swaying. This was followed by a loss of mental sharpness and trouble focusing their vision.

The volunteers were wrapped for only about 2 minutes, but the point was made: Plastic materials can unbalance our subtle bodies.

The remedy, after unwrapping the volunteers, was to have them simply say aloud:

"With my spirit, I accept Divine Love and ask that my body be charged and balanced."

Immediately, both volunteers announced that all discomfort had left and they were returned to a normal condition!

FOR THE TEST APPLICATIONS IN THIS CHAPTER, PLEASE USE THE FINGER DOUSING TECHNIQUE TO MEASURE.

Supplement Testing

A regular routine for me is verifying what vitamins and supplements I need and the dosage required for each to maintain good health.

I suggest you develop a similar testing habit to determine:

1. If you need the supplement being tested.

2. If the supplement will work properly with your other supplements or medications.

3. The correct dosage to take for each.

First, hold a supplement in the hand forming the test ring. Close your other fingers over the test supplement to hold it. Test by asking:

"Do I need this supplement?"

If the answer is NO, do not take the supplement. If the answer is YES, proceed to the next step.

Place all other supplements and daily medications in a small glass with the test supplement. Then hold the glass in the hand forming the test ring and ask:

"Is this supplement safe to take with my other supplements and medications?"

If the answer is YES, the correct daily dosage needs to be determined. If the answer is NO, then that supplement must be taken at a different time and not with the other products. You need to test further to determine what dosage to take and when.

In both cases, to establish the daily dosage required:

Set the glass down.

Hold the test supplement in the hand forming the test ring. You may need to repeat this test several times, increasing the dosage to determine the correct level.

Suppose you have a 100mg tablet and you suspect your body requires 400mg per day, but you do not know for certain; that is what you are testing to learn. Start with the lowest dosage, test for that, then if a larger dosage is required, test for the next increment. Ask:

"Should I take 100mg or more per day of this supplement?"

In this example, you should be getting a YES, which means that the dosage is 100mg or more. We said that this was a test case, so you need to keep testing to find the correct level. Ask:

"Should I take 200mg or more per day of this supplement?"

Again, you should be getting a YES, but you don't yet know if you've reached the correct limit, so test again. Ask:

"Should I take 300mg or more per day of this supplement?"

The answer should be a YES, but again you are not sure if you've reached the limit. Ask:

"Should I take 400mg or more per day of this supplement?"

Again, you get a YES, but since you don't know if this is the correct dosage, test for the next highest dosage. Ask:

"Should I take 500mg or more per day of this supplement?"

This time the test answer should yield a NO, which means that you reached the limit at 400mg; that is the dosage you should be taking. To continue: You are holding a 100mg tablet and you need to know how many to take at one time. Ask:

"Should I take two tablets with my morning meal?"

If the answer is YES, you are nearly finished evaluating frequency. Since most supplements and medications are distributed throughout the day, you might want to find out when you should take the other 200mg by asking:

"Should I take 200mg with my evening meal?"

I would expect that you would get a YES, which means you should take 200mg at breakfast time and 200mg at suppertime. However, if the answer was NO, you would need to ask a question to properly split the frequency. You might ask:

"Should I take 100mg at midday?

If the answer is YES, you need to know when

to take the remaining 100mg. You might test by asking the following until you receive a YES:

"Should I take a total of 200mg at midday?" NO

"Should I take 100mg later in the evening?" NO

"Should I take 100mg at suppertime?" YES

By testing correctly you learned exactly when you should be taking your supplement. The schedule is: 200mg at breakfast time, 100mg at midday, and 100mg at suppertime.

This may seem to be an extreme level of detail, but remember that you are testing your supplement against *all* your other supplements and medications. Therefore, if you receive what appears to be a strange answer, it means that your test supplement may be interacting with one or more of your other supplements or your medications.

But testing may not be finished! Some supplements and medications are to be taken on an empty stomach, perhaps an hour before eating or several hours afterwards. You should closely read and follow the instructions for supplements and medications.

The chapter on medications gives examples of how side effects develop. You certainly want to prevent medication and/or supplement interactions that could become harmful.

It is important to determine the exact dosage and frequency required by your body. Do not hesitate to test; your body will not lie.

Foods

Are you concerned about particular foods? Perhaps you ate a piece of cheese and now your stomach feels queasy. Why not test it? Hold a small piece of the cheese in your hand

and ask:

"Should I eat this type of cheese?"

If the answer is NO, you will know to avoid that type of cheese in the future.

Perhaps the answer is YES, but you wonder what made you queasy; you need to ask more specific questions until you can ascertain what the problem really is. You might ask:

"Is this cheese responsible for making my stomach queasy?"

If the answer is NO, then something that you ate with the cheese, e.g., a flavored cracker, may be upsetting your stomach.

If the answer is YES, it means that it is still okay to eat the cheese, but not with something else. Perhaps the cheese reacted with something previously eaten; you might consider eating less cheese by testing for how much your body can handle or testing for conflicts with other foods.

You know this is the *correct approach* because when you first tested, it was okay to eat the cheese, but the second test revealed that the cheese eaten with something else made you feel unwell.

Do you see the many ways YOU can be a spiritual scientist in your approach to foods, supplements, and medications?

Prescription Testing

The medicine chapter explained how side effects can exist and develop based upon your personal history.

With the luxury of time, you can test any medication, either currently being taken or being recommended, against unknown old compounds already present in your system.

Test medications in the same manner as supplements. Medications are more complex to test, but it is doable. Some medications must be taken with food, others on an empty stomach, and some should not be taken with certain other things such as potassium or calcium.

Test Method

You want to know whether a medication being recommended to you is safe to take in your present condition, without exposing you to negative side effects or discomfort. Put all your medications and supplements into a small glass that you can hold. If you want to know whether to take them all together or not, you might ask:

"Should I take all these tablets together at the same time?"

If the answer is YES, you may take them all together. However, if the answer is NO, you need to test further to determine how you should be taking that medication. It may be difficult to cover all potential combinations, but it would be prudent to investigate as many test options as possible. Again, closely read and follow the medical instructions.

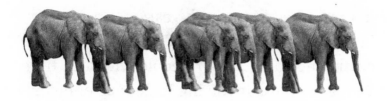

Dynamic Reality:
The Divine Love
Addiction Healing Program

From the 2016 Surgeon General's Report on Alcohol, Drugs and Health:

"Alcohol and drug misuse and related substance use disorders affect millions of Americans and impose enormous costs on our society. In 2015, 66.7 million people in the United States reported binge drinking in the past month and 27.1 million people were current users of illicit drugs or misused prescription drugs."

"Alcohol misuse contributes to 88,000 deaths

in the United States each year; . . . In addition, in 2014 there were 47,055 drug overdose deaths including 28,647 people who died from a drug overdose involving some type of opioid, including prescription pain relievers and heroin. . ."

"Only about 1 in 10 people with a substance use disorder receive any type of specialty treatment."

What Is Needed For Successful Rehabilitation?

Three humane objectives must be met for lasting recovery:

1. Detox the body without incurring unnecessary pain.

2. Heal any chemical damage to the body or brain.

3. Release and heal all underlying causes of the addiction.

Inpatient and outpatient detox centers usually provide medical treatments and safe environments. Yet, even when withdrawal drugs are provided, detox can be painful.

I am not aware of any medical technology to treat chemical damage; it is doubtful that researchers will find a general solution because of the *chemical soup* that is in most bodies. Remember that drugs and toxins from any source can react in the body and form other compounds capable of destroying cells and neural circuits in the brain.

The removal of underlying causes may require years of therapy when normal medical conventions are followed. This is not viable for several reasons:

Millions of people would need therapy;

Therapy is seldom effective for short-term participants;

And lastly, there aren't enough qualified therapists willing to work in this field.

Available Treatments

Many excellent private treatment facilities assist people in breaking their addictions to drugs and alcohol. Private facilities offer the addicted person access to many services including: managed drug withdrawal, medication programs, managed exercise programs, extensive psychological counseling, access to good food, and pleasant surroundings. The length of stay can be several months.

However, these facilities tend to be expensive; costs are not always covered by insurance, and these facilities may be unavailable to people without insurance.

Meet the Elephant in the Room

The duration of state-funded and most county-funded rehabilitation programs is typically 28 days. However, the failure rate is close to 70% for people enrolled in these rehab programs. Some reasons for that high failure rate:

Some people have no desire to end their addictions; they are only in a rehab program because it was court ordered.

The demand for more drugs can be created when brain chemistry has been altered.

People who do want help may not receive enough psychological counseling to get to the heart of their problems.

The Bottom Line

Private or public facilities are able to detox people.

Once released from a rehab center, addicts are often encouraged to participate in ongoing 12-Step Programs where the group provides follow-on mutual support.

Dynamic Realities and Divine Love Healing

For people who believe in a higher power or Creator, these programs can be effective. For those who do not believe in a higher power, the Programs may have spotty results.

People in recovery often have a fear that they will relapse and fall back into their addiction habits. Even after 5 to 7 years, a person driven by that fear will often relapse.

Medical researchers have written much about drug addiction and we are familiar with the notion that "drugs can fry the brain." Unfortunately, no prescription drug programs correct brain damage; the degree of damage and mixtures of drugs are usually unknown.

When sufficient counseling is not provided, the underlying causes of addiction are not cleared. This *elephant in the room* "time bomb" can manifest in violence and/or re-addiction.

Why Our Program?

Although we have had many successes helping individuals recover from drug and alcohol addictions over the past 30 years, we did not present addiction healing and recovery to the general public until recently.

With increased worldwide concern about addiction problems, we recognized that a group program needed to be introduced to handle the millions of people currently addicted. Technology and dollars alone are incapable of solving these problems in the short term.

Our Approach

We wanted to have a program that could be used with Divine Love to help reduce the growing drug addiction problem. The Program did not depend upon a participant's prior knowledge of Divine Love healing. We provided only basic instruction so as not to complicate the study.

Dynamic Realities and Divine Love Healing

We initiated a proof-of-concept spiritual research program by placing into the mass consciousness field a modified *At Oneness Healing System Advanced Protocol* to address drug and alcohol abuse. In March 2017, we invited people on our mailing list to participate in our free spiritual *Divine Love Addiction Healing Program* for alcohol and drug addictions.

Enrollment was between April 1 and June 15; the Program ran from April through August 2017. Participants connected to the *Advanced Protocol* by saying a Healing Statement once per day.

Survey Questions

We asked each enrolled person to answer a series of survey questions:

1. Do you believe that the Creator cares about you and is making, or has made, you well?

2. Do you accept the healing of your addiction?

3. Please describe your experience 24 hours after submitting your registration for this program.

4. As of today, do you feel a need/desire to continue your addiction?

5. How many days after starting this Program, did you stop taking the drugs or alcohol related to your addiction?

6. If you have experienced complete detox, please describe your physical and emotional feelings.

7. Do you believe that your healing is complete?

8. Do you believe that the root cause(s) of your addiction are completely healed?

9. If you don't believe your healing for addiction is complete, what do you think is preventing healing?

We repeated this survey two additional times to evaluate progress over a three-week period.

People were quick to acknowledge that detox took place without pain, a major accomplishment! They also reported improved mental clarity, which was obvious as they became more articulate with subsequent surveys.

Most people wanted to understand why they had previously been unable to break the addiction cycle. I believe this occurs because dopamine and other chemicals produced in the brain create an overwhelming need that can only be satisfied by more drugs. We believe complete recovery requires the treatment of chemical damage and the underlying causes of the addiction.

In my experience, the only lasting solution to alcohol and drug addiction is spiritual healing with Divine Love, when the three healing objectives are achieved: detoxing without more drugs, healing of chemical damage, and releasing and healing all underlying causes of addiction.

Results – Removing Elephants From The Room

At the end of August 2017, we closely examined the reports from 50 program participants. 86% of survey respondents reported success for the Divine Love Addiction Healing Program in less than a week! 14% did not achieve their goals because they believed they needed to continue their addictions to remain social. Lost to follow-up were 67 program participants who did not respond to survey requests.

This amazing result is a Dynamic Reality because traditional 28-day residential rehab programs:

Take about a week to detox with medications designed to lessen withdrawal.

Cannot heal chemical damage, and,

Lack the residence time to comprehensively release the underlying causes of addiction.

Although some might question how an addict can report objectively, without oversight by professionals trained in psychology or psychiatry, the results speak for themselves. The healing process is effective.

About Our Third Objective: Removal of Underlying Causes

We've been told by therapists that people finishing a 28-day rehab/detox program fall into one of two categories:

The recovering addict who fails and resumes the addiction within about a two-week period following their rehab facility release.

The recovering addict who joins group therapy such as a 12-Step Program. People in those programs receive spiritual guidance to correct behavior and develop new healthy habits. Some people succeed; others do not.

Our Program has not run long enough to test whether or not people in recovery will remain completely free beyond the 5 to 7 year time frame. However, in my experience working directly with people over the last 30 years, I do not know of one person who resumed a past addiction.

The Future of the Drug and Alcohol Addiction Program

When I realized the magnitude of the training program required to teach this *Advanced Protocol*, the limitations were obvious. Not enough people could be reached in a reasonable time frame. There would also be push back from institutions with established programs. And, we'd need to raise considerable funds to implement our program. Three other problems needed to be addressed:

1. There needed to be an automatic registration

mechanism to admit people into a worldwide Program. The registration would accept people who were motivated to be well, and filter out those who were not. We certainly did not feel comfortable putting any restraints on registration, but we saw in the lost to follow-up numbers that people apparently registered who were less committed.

2. Some people assigned to court-ordered rehab are not interested in participating in a county- or state-managed program.

3. Because some people in our program were lost to follow-up, future results could be criticized. (Our greater concern, however, is that those people find a solution for their addictions.)

Since we were unable to resolve these three problems, we decided to place into the energy field of the mass consciousness a second modified *At Oneness Healing System Advanced Protocol.* This modified *Protocol* is used for the Divine Love Addiction Healing Program. We asked the Creator's Angels to take over the worldwide administration and expansion of this Program. And they did!

People desiring admission to this Angel-led program may apply using their spiritual intention. Then an Angel asks an individual's internal spirit if that individual is to be part of the Program. If the answer is YES, the individual is admitted to the program and enjoys the benefits as the program proceeds. If the answer is NO, the individual is not admitted to the program.

By keeping the *Advanced Protocol* in the mass consciousness field, we are able to simplify *Protocol* use in several ways:

All the "pop-ups" normally encountered are automatically dissolved with deep breathing; a participant does not have to do anything more to remove the "pop-ups."

Dynamic Realities and Divine Love Healing

A participant remains automatically connected to all the Petitions in the Advanced Protocol.

The participant does not say Petitions.

In the months and years ahead, watch for a significant decrease in overdose deaths and more reports of unexplained complete healing. Then you will better understand the spiritual truth of the Creator's Divine Love.

This Program may be your best example of a Dynamic Reality; it allows you and others to help correct problems that are too widespread and/or too costly to be addressed by existing therapies.

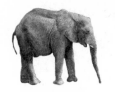 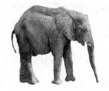 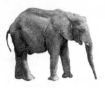

Dynamic Reality:
Alzheimer's
Divine Love Healing Program

Alzheimer's is the sixth leading cause of death in the Unoted States.

Alzheimer's disease has no conventional medical treatment for both *cause* and *effect*. Also, the costs to maintain Alzheimer's patients can be overwhelming.

In the United States, a few federally approved medictions are used to treat Alzheimer's and perhaps slow its progression, but none heal the *cause* of Alzheimer's.

Dynamic Realities and Divine Love Healing

It has been predicted that the number of people with Alzheimer's will double to 10 million in the United States within a few years. Residential care facilities for Alzheimer's patients are in short supply and financial aid is often not available. Families are left with few options: provide safety-oriented caregiving in homes or in special wards of nursing homes or assisted living facilities.

Having dealt with many different illnesses, we know that our Divine Love *At Oneness Healing System Advanced Protocol* corrects both *symptoms* AND *underlying causes.*

On June 26, 2017, using a modified *At Oneness Healing System Advanced Protocol* placed into the mass consciousness, we initiated a free spiritual research Alzheimer's Divine Love Healing Program.

Participation was limited to individuals on our mailing list and their designated loved ones. Cognitive patients were given a Healing

Statement from the *Advanced Protocol* to recite one time daily, without further instructions. When a family member or caregiver enrolled a patient who had little or no cognitive function, the caregiver or a volunteer would say the necessary Healing Statement on behalf of the patient.

Many who applied for help did not have a background in our teachings, webinars, or books. To help individuals develop confidence in our spiritual research Program, we included the following information in our Program Announcement:

Program Announcement Excerpts

We provided interested parties with this five-component program:

1. What is Divine Love and How Does It Work?

Divine Love is the Creator's Love, God's Love,

and is an energy force that actually changes the human condition. Divine Love removes energetic disturbances and restores the human body to a state wherein the cells can once again function properly. That effect is called spiritual healing and it requires only two things from a participant:

A belief in God, the Creator of the universe, or other higher power, and

A sincere desire to change to a state of wellness.

2. How the Alzheimer's Divine Love Healing Program Works

Divine Love healing functions in the same manner for everyone. Harmful energy, biological toxins and chemical toxins enter the brain and interfere with brain cells, causing the cells to malfunction. Because Divine Love heals all conditions, the brain can heal.

3. Our Expectations for You

Alzheimer's severity is described clinically by seven stages of mental and physical deterioration. We accept people from any stage into this research Program because Divine Love is not limited.

With our more than 30 years' experience with Divine Love spiritual healing, we expect that you can achieve positive results with this Program, according to the Creator's will.

Our intentions for this spiritual healing research Program are:

To show that Alzheimer's can be healed with Divine Love utilizing our *At Oneness Healing System Advanced Protocol.*

To help establish a better understanding of Divine Love as a healing energy to achieve healthcare solutions.

4. Features and Benefits

The Creator manages each participant's overall healing process.

Physical contact with participants is unneeded.

Divine Love spiritual healing can correct chemical deterioration in the brain, thus restoring the participant.

A participant continues normal activities while Divine Love spiritual healing operates in the background.

A participant says aloud a single Healing Statement daily. If the participant cannot say the Healing Statement, a caregiver, relative, or friend may act as proxy and say the Healing Statement from any location.

This is a spiritual research Program.

5. Reporting

We ask that the participant or caregiver report progress via a weekly status report. We will email all requests for status reports. Personal identities and all information reported are held in strict confidence.

Alzheimer's Report Survey

The 2017 survey consisted of this simple non-invasive question:

What changes did you observe in the participant this week?

The caregivers were forthcoming, with many sharing information about other conditions of their participants.

Alzheimer Program Results

The findings from this Program as of February 26, 2018:

Of the 25 participants who responded to our survey, most reported progress recovering from this illness.

44% reported major improvement in cognitive function, speech and calmness; 20% reported slight improvement and progress.

36% reported no change or a continued decline in cognitive function. 29 participants were lost to follow-up.

Report Analysis

The weekly reports mentioned behavioral and cognitive swings in Alzheimer's patients who were often sedated by medications. One week a report would indicate a patient's becoming more alert and cognitive. The next week's report might indicate a decline in alertness or cognitive function because of medications or other unspecified causes.

Since we know that Divine Love can overcome

negative side effects, there seem to be only two issues frustrating healing:

1. The personal desire of the patient. Some reports indicated that the patients demonstrated no interest in becoming well, perhaps due to their loss of cognition.

2. Many of the participants in this Program also had complicating issues such as heart disease, broken bones, breathing disorders, systemic infections and cancer. Additional healing time is required in cases of life-threatening illnesses before the Alzheimer's can be addressed.

Advanced Protocol Modifications for Alzheimer's Healing

When the Advanced Protocol was originally set up to run automatically in the mass consciousness, the symptom used in the Healing Statement was "brain damage."

Dynamic Realities and Divine Love Healing

People reporting Alzheimer improvement had no other major health issues, but when we learned that many of our Alzheimer Program participants had additional severe health problems frustrating their healing, we changed the Healing Statement symptom to "brain and body" to achieve a more complete healing, according to the Creator's will.

We also adjusted the Healing Statement to run automatically with or without any caregiver support.

Every participant should have the opportunity to heal. Therefore, we decided to continue this program and asked the Creator's Angels to manage the Program using the same criteria as used in the Divine Love Addiction Healing Program. Time will tell how effective this free healing Program is!

Epilogue

After learning how these healing systems were developed and applied, you should be convinced that Divine Love is a real energy force, a Dynamic Reality. Divine Love can be used for self-healing and does not conflict with conventional medicine.

When we ask for it, information comes to us from the Divine, but that information must be interpreted and properly applied. This is the Dynamic Reality that makes spiritual healing possible.

If you are in the healthcare profession, you may want to build your own *Advanced Protocol* from the information contained in this book. Then apply it in your practice.

My first objective was to keep people continuously connected to the energy of Divine Love. That objective has been achieved with the *Advanced Protocol*.

My second objective was to provide the *Advanced Protocol* to those who may never read this book or take a webinar. That objective was achieved by placing the *Advanced Protocol* into the mass consciousness and then using it successfully for the *Divine Love Addiction Healing Program*.

Many health problems in the world today cannot be solved by the application of conventional medical solutions. Even when solutions exist, often the side effects introduce additional issues and risks. *These problems are all "elephants in the room" that need to be removed!*

On the other hand, because we now have

experience working with many different illnesses, it would seem natural to include the *Advanced Protocol* as part of everyone's health recovery and maintenance program.

The *Advanced Protocol* worked so well in the mass consciousness that we have also placed a general-purpose *Advanced Protocol* into the mass consciousness.

The 2018 Advanced Protocol Healing Statement Webinars

For those of you who do NOT want to build your own Advanced Protocol, I suggest you attend one of our 2018 and beyond Healing Statement Webinars. During the Webinar you will learn how to access and use the mass consciousness-based *Advanced Protocol.* You will also learn to remove all pop-ups automatically with a single Healing Statement.

Then you will be able to share the modified *Advanced Protocol* and modified Healing Statement information with your family and friends.

My Wish for You

After reading this book you can see that the development and testing of these concepts has taken me on a long enlightening journey. Remember that all information in this book can be used to complement conventional medical practices.

I sincerely hope you will take full advantage of this opportunity to restore your health and live a more meaningful life with Divine Love.

Robert G. Fritchie
March 2018

Appendix

Many people have been given conflicting definitions of God, the Creator of the universe.

In 1947, James Dillet Freeman, anguished by the approaching death of his wife, called out to God for help. The message he received from God was published as a poem and has been shared with people all over the world.

This poem touched my heart. Perhaps it will touch yours as well.

I AM THERE
by
James Dillet Freeman

Do you need Me?
I am there.

You cannot see Me, yet I am the light you see by.
You cannot hear Me, yet I speak through your voice.
You cannot feel Me, yet I am the power at work in
your hands.

I am at work, though you do not understand My ways.
I am at work, though you do not recognize My works.
I am not strange visions. I am not mysteries.

Only in absolute stillness, beyond self, can you know
Me as I am, and then but as a feeling and a faith.
Yet I am there. Yet I hear. Yet I answer.

When you need Me, I am there.
Even if you deny Me, I am there.
Even when you feel most alone, I am there.
Even in your fears, I am there.
Even in your pain, I am there.

Removing Elephants from the Room

I am there when you pray and when you do not pray.
I am in you, and you are in Me.

Only in your mind can you feel separate from Me, for
only in your mind are the mists of "yours" and "mine."
Yet only with your mind can you know Me and
experience Me.

Empty your heart of empty fears.
When you get yourself out of the way, I am there.

You can of yourself do nothing, but I can do all.
And I am in all.
Though you may not see the good, good is there, for I
am there.

I am there because I have to be, because I am.
Only in Me does the world have meaning;
Only out of Me does the world take form;
Only because of Me does the world go forward.

I am the law on which the movement of the stars and
the growth of living cells are founded.

I am the love that is the law's fulfilling.
I am assurance.
I am peace.
I am oneness.

Dynamic Realities and Divine Love Healing

I am the law that you can live by.
I am the love that you can cling to.
I am your assurance.
I am your peace.
I am one with you.
I am.

Though you fail to find Me, I do not fail you.
Though your faith in Me is unsure, My faith in you
never wavers,

Because I know you, because I love you.
Beloved, I am there.